D1756912

This book is to be returned on or before
the last date stamped below.

New Aspects of Cochlear Mechanics and Inner Ear Pathophysiology

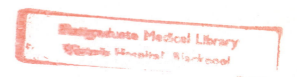

Advances in Oto-Rhino-Laryngology

Vol. 44

Series Editor
C.R. Pfaltz, Basel

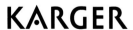

Basel · München · Paris · London · New York · New Delhi · Bangkok · Singapore · Tokyo · Sydney

New Aspects of Cochlear Mechanics and Inner Ear Pathophysiology

Volume Editor
C.R. Pfaltz, Basel

59 figures and 16 tables, 1990

KARGER

Basel · München · Paris · London · New York · New Delhi · Bangkok · Singapore · Tokyo · Sydney

Advances in Oto-Rhino-Laryngology

Library of Congress Catologing-in-Publication Data
New aspects of cochlear mechanics and inner ear pathophysiology/
volume editor, C.R. Pfaltz.
(Advances in oto-rhino-laryngology; vol. 44)
Includes bibliographical references.
1. Labyrinth (Ear) – Effect of drugs on.   2. Ototoxic agents – Physiological effect.
3. Diuretics – Toxicology.   4. Cochlea – Physiology.   5. Physiology, Experimental.
I. Pfaltz, C.R. (Carl Rudolf)   II. Series.
[DNLM: 1. Acoustic Stimulation.   2. Cochlea – drug effects.
3. Cochlea – physiology.
ISBN 3-8055-5020-0

Bibliographic Indices
This publication is listed in bibliographic services, including Current Contents® and Index Medicus.

Drug Dosage
The authors and the publisher have exerted every effort to ensure that drug selection and dosage set forth in this text are in accord with current recommendations and practice at the time of publication. However, in view of ongoing research, changes in government regulations and the constant flow of information relating to drug therapy and drug reactions, the reader is urged to check the package insert for each drug for any change in indications and dosage and for added warnings and precautions. This is particularly important when the recommended agent is a new and/or infrequently employed drug.

© Copyright 1990 by S. Karger AG, P.O. Box, CH–4009 Basel (Switzerland)
Printed in Switzerland by Thür AG Offsetdruck, Pratteln
ISBN 3–8055–5020–0

Contents

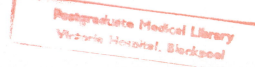

Contents

Ototoxicity of Loop Diuretics. Morphological and Electrophysiological Examinations in Animal Experiments

Christian Peter Hommerich, Düsseldorf 92

Preface

Inner ear sensitivity to toxic side effects of various drugs has been known for more than a century. According to J. E. Hawkins, ototoxicity is "the tendency of certain therapeutic agents and other chemical substances to cause functional impairment and cellular degeneration of the tissues of the inner ear, and especially of the end organs and neurons of the cochlear and vestibular divisions of the eighth cranial nerve".

The ototoxic effect of aminoglycosides has been studied very carefully since it became evident, shortly after its use in humans (1945), that it could produce deafness and balance disorders. Heretofore little was known about the ototoxic effects of "loop inhibiting" diuretics such as ethacrynic acid and furosemide. Since the first published report about immediate but reversible sensorineural hearing loss combined with vestibular symptoms following intravenous administration of ethacrynic acid, many years passed until the underlying pathophysiologic mechanisms were clarified to some extent. Fundamental questions still remain open, but C. Hommerich makes a successful attempt to present an overview on the current understanding of ototoxicity resulting from use of loop diuretics and to clarify prevailing concepts of endolymph production in the cochlea.

New aspects of cochlear mechanics followed the discovery by Kemp that the cochlea not only receives sounds, but also produces acoustic energy referred to as *acoustic emissions*. R. Probst presents an overview on this finding based on the results of personal experimental studies in animals and humans and discusses the biological significance of this phenomenon. Moreover, he emphasizes the clinical significance of otoacoustic emissions which now permit examination and monitoring of basic cochlear mechanisms in an objective and noninvasive way.

C. R. Pfaltz, Basel

Pfaltz CR (ed): New Aspects of Cochlear Mechanics and Inner Ear Pathophysiology.
Adv Otorhinolaryngol. Basel, Karger, 1990, vol 44, pp 1–91

Otoacoustic Emissions: An Overview

R. Probst

Department of Otorhinolaryngology, Kantonsspital, University of Basel,
Basel, Switzerland

1. Introduction

The idea of cochlear function has undergone fundamental changes in the past decade. A multitude of morphological, physiological, psychoacoustical, and modeling studies have substantially contributed to this progress. Several recent reviews [Allen, 1985; Dallos, 1985; Hudspeth, 1985a, b; Pickles, 1985; Lim, 1986; Lippe, 1986; Klinke, 1987; Zenner and Gitter, 1987] provide summaries of these findings and of the new concepts evolving from them.

One of the recent discoveries contributing substantially to the new understanding of cochlear function was the demonstration that the cochlea does not only receive sounds, but can also produce acoustic energy. Though Gold [1948] postulated such sounds as long ago as 1948, they were only first detected 30 years later by Kemp [1978]. He demonstrated that sound produced by the cochlea can be recorded in the ear canal with special methods. Today, these sounds are generally called otoacoustic emissions (OAE).

The discovery of OAE was important for several reasons. One of them was that the presence of active biophysical mechanisms within the cochlea became likely. Most probably, the cochlea does not only passively receive acoustic energy, but it actively amplifies certain sounds producing oscillations of its own. New mathematical or physical models of the cochlea had to consider these properties. Moreover, anatomical structures capable of active and rapid oscillations had to be designated or discovered. This necessity led to new interpretations of many findings from microscopic or ultrastructural anatomical studies. At the same time, some findings from physiological studies, either newly discovered or known for many years, could be explained with a new approach.

Another reason for the importance of OAE was the possibility to study mechanical aspects of cochlear function in a noninvasive and objective way [Kemp, 1988]. The cochlea could be studied 'from another side', with new methods not dependent on nerve action potentials and with a direct connection to its mechanical function. OAE allow repeated measures of cochlear functions over long time periods without interference with the physiological mode of operation.

The possible clinical importance of OAE is in this noninvasive and direct window to the cochlea. Objective information about preneural, mechanical elements of the cochlea can be obtained clinically with the help of OAE. The majority of peripheral hearing losses, such as noise induced or hereditary hearing losses, have their origin in these elements. Objective methods presently in clinical use do not measure responses of these elements directly. While evoked potentials rely on nerve responses following these elements, the examination of the stapedial reflex tests a multineuron event. Therefore, OAE may very well supplement these clinical methods.

Our understanding of OAE, their phenomenology, interrelations among different forms of OAE, and relation to pathology has improved substantially in the decade since Kemp's [1978] discovery. However, there are many open questions and a comprehensive understanding of the generation of OAE is still lacking. Similarly, the use of OAE as a clinical test is still impeded by the lack of knowledge about many of their aspects. Therefore, this overview will not give a definitive statement about OAE. The aim of this review is to summarize the knowledge about the different forms of OAE, to define the state of the art, and to make some speculations about the future use of OAE and their importance in clinical otology.

2. Definition and General Remarks

2.1. Classes of Otoacoustic Emissions

Any sound that is produced by the cochlea and that can be recorded in the ear canal is defined as an OAE. This definition implies a known cochlear origin of these sounds. Before discussing the evidence indicating this origin, several interrelated classes of OAE will be distinguished. One type is spontaneoulsy present without external stimulation. Other classes of emissions are evoked by different kinds of acoustic stimulation. They can be further divided into three classes according to the particular type of stimulation that evokes them. Table 1 lists these four classes of OAE along with the abbreviations used in this overview. Although previously given different names, these four classes are uniformly recognized in the literature. A summary of these names along with a short description of the classes will be given first.

(1) The first class consists of narrowband signals that can be measured in the absence of deliberate acoustic stimulation. These emissions are

Table 1. Classes of OAE

1. Spontaneous OAE	SOAE
2. Transiently evoked OAE	TEOAE
3. Stimulus-frequency OAE	SFOAE
4. OAE of distortion products	DPOAE

generally called 'spontaneous otoacoustic emissions' (SOAE). They are stationary signals that can be recorded over long time periods.

(2) The second class of emissions, evoked by transient stimulations, is the type first described by Kemp [1978]. He initally called them 'stimulated acoustic emissions'. These emissions can be recorded by a time averaging procedure after a short acoustic stimulation such as a click. Kemp referred to these emissions in later studies as 'evoked cochlear mechanical responses' [1979a] or as 'echoes' [1980, 1982]. Zwicker [1983a] used the term 'delayed evoked otoacoustic emissions' because of their typical occurrence after the stimulus. Other investigators called these emissions 'Kemp echoes' [Wit et al., 1981] or simply 'evoked emissions' [Rutten, 1980a; Johnsen and Elberling, 1982a, b].

Despite the many terms already existing, the expression 'transiently evoked otoacoustic emission' (TEOAE) is preferred here, since the distinction of the different classes of OAE relies on the type of stimulation. The characteristic stimulation for these emissions is transient. Moreover, the other expressions are somewhat imprecise, since all types of OAE with the exception of SOAE occur after stimulation, they all are mechanical responses of the cochlea, and many of them show a certain latency. In addition, the term 'echo' may be misleading, since echoes are purely passive events and active elements are likely to be involved in the generation of OAE.

(3) An acoustic stimulation with low-level constant tones can lead to the generation of additional acoustic energy from the cochlea at the frequency of stimulation. Therefore, these emissions were called 'stimulus-frequency otoacoustic emissions' (SFOAE) [Kemp and Chum, 1980a]. Schloth [1982] and Zwicker and Schloth [1984] used the term 'synchronously evoked otoacoustic emissions'. Since OAE of distortion products are also evoked synchronously, the term 'stimulus-frequency emissions' will be used here.

(4) Acoustic distortion products (DP) are generated by nonlinear elements during acoustic stimulation and are tones with frequencies other than those of the stimuli. The frequency of the DP is related to the primary stimulus frequencies by exact mathematical expressions. For example, harmonic distortions are a full multiple of the frequency of the stimulus. A

bitonal stimulation can elicit many different DP, the so-called 'intermodulation products'. The cochlea as a nonlinear system creates such DP, some of
which can be detected as OAE in the ear canal. They are called 'distortion
product OAE' (DPOAE) [Kemp, 1979a].

These four classes of OAE will be described separately and in more
detail in later sections. First, however, some aspects common to all classes
of OAE will be described.

2.2. Cochlear Origin

The discovery of OAE was first met with much scepticism [Wilson,
1984]. These emissions were believed to be an artifact, possibly related to
the middle ear. Therefore, many different experiments were conducted with
the aim of proving the cochlear origin of OAE. Today, the cochlear
generation of OAE is well documented and generally accepted. Most of the
evidence supporting this will be discussed along with separate descriptions
of the different classes of OAE. Some of the most important findings
pointing to a cochlear origin are compiled in the following paragraphs. The
pertinent references are summarized without detailed discussion, sometimes
in tables.

2.2.1. Noise Exposure. All four types of OAE can be influenced by
acoustic overstimulation. Amplitudes are reduced as a first effect. Table 2
summarizes the most important references. While the findings in human ears
were based on relatively short exposures inducing temporary threshold shifts
(TTS), experiments in animals used generally longer exposures inducing
more definite cochlear damage. The most thoroughly studied OAE in this
respect are the DPOAE, though in many studies other experimental aims
than the demonstration of the cochlear origin were important.

2.2.2. Suppression. The amplitude of an OAE can be reduced by
stimulation with additional tones and the amount of suppression is dependent on the frequency and intensity of the suppressing tone. The study of
suppression contours of OAE revealed that they were highly tuned and
similar to those found in single nerve fiber studies. Therefore, the generation of OAE is related to tuned elements, generally believed to be localized
in the cochlea. Again, references are summarized in table 3.

2.2.3. Ototoxic Drugs. Additional evidence pointing to the cochlear
origin of OAE comes from studies with ototoxic drugs. Such drugs are
toxic to cochlear structures and their ingestion was shown to lead to a
reduction or elimination of OAE amplitudes. The diuretics furosemide and
ethacryne acid were studied in primates [Anderson and Kemp, 1979;

Table 2. Synopsis of references concerning noise exposure and OAE

	Human	Animal
SOAE	Norton et al. [1986, 1987] Dear et al. [1986]	Evans et al. [1981]
TEOAE	Kemp [1981, 1982, 1986] Anderson [1980]	Anderson and Kemp [1979] Wilson and Evans [1983]
SFOAE	–	Kössl and Vater [1985]
DPOAE	–	Kim et al. [1980] Siegel and Kim [1982a] Zurek et al. [1982] Schmiedt and Addy [1982] Rosowski et al. [1984b] Dolan and Abbas [1985a, b] Schmiedt [1986a] Wiederhold et al. [1986] Stainbeck et al. [1987] Lonsbury-Martin et al. [1987] Martin et al. [1987a]

Table 3. Synopsis of references concerning suppression of OAE

	Human	Animal
SOAE	Zurek [1981] Wilson [1980a] Wilson and Sutton [1981] Schloth [1982] Ruggero et al. [1983] Rabinowitz and Widin [1984] Dallmayr [1985] Rebillard et al. [1987] Bargones and Burns [1988] Frick and Matthies [1988]	Evans et al. [1981] Clark et al. [1984] Ruggero et al. [1984] Martin et al. [1988]
TEOAE	Kemp [1979a] Wit and Ritsma [1979] Wilson and Sutton [1981] Wit et al. [1981] Schloth [1982]	–
SFOAE	Kemp and Chum [1980a] Dallmayr [1987]	Manley et al. [1987]
DPOAE	Brown and Kemp [1984]	Brown and Kemp [1984] Kemp and Brown [1984] Martin et al. [1987a]

Anderson, 1980], in gerbils [Kemp and Brown, 1984], and in cats [Wilson and Evans, 1983].

The effect of aspirin, a drug with reversible ototoxicity [McFadden et al., 1984], was tested in animals and human subjects. Studies in humans revealed that SOAE were reduced or abolished by aspirin administration [McFadden and Plattsmier, 1984]. Transiently evoked emission or SFOAE were also affected, though less than SOAE [Johnsen and Elberling, 1982a; Long et al., 1986; Long and Tubis, 1988]. Figure 1 shows an example of the influence of aspirin on a short-lasting TEOAE. Similar effects were found for SOAE and SFOAE in the rhesus monkey [Martin et al., 1988]. However, DPOAE were unchanged during aspirin administration in this monkey. A dissociation between the effect of aspirin on SOAE and on DPOAE was also found for human subjects [Wier et al., 1988]. Important differences in the assumed generation mechanisms of SOAE or SFOAE and DPOAE may be partially responsible for these different effects of aspirin.

2.2.4. Hypoxia. A SOAE [Evans et al., 1981] and TEOAE [Zwicker and Manley, 1981] could be abolished promptly and reversibly by hypoxia in guinea pigs. Anoxia or hypoxia also led to the reduction of DPOAE amplitudes, which were studied in different species of laboratory animals [Kim et al., 1980; Schmied and Adams, 1981; Kemp and Brown, 1984; Horner et al., 1985; Wiederhold et al., 1986; Lonsbury-Martin et al., 1987]. However, remarkable differences in the postmortem time course were found in these studies. Details will be discussed together with the properties of DPOAE.

The reduction or abolition of OAE under hypoxic conditions point to a metabolic dependent generation of these emissions not compatible with an origin within the middle ear.

2.2.5. Hearing Loss. Emissions, such as TEOAE or SOAE, are generally undetectable if hearing losses of more than 25–30 dB HL are present. Kemp [1978] pointed out this fact in his first description of TEOAE. This finding is frequency specific, i.e. no TEOAE may be found in frequency regions where the hearing loss is greater than 30 dB, along with still present TEOAE or SOAE in other frequency regions in the same ear where the hearing threshold is relatively normal [Rutten, 1980a; Zurek, 1981; Kemp et al., 1986; Probst et al., 1987]. These two findings, dependence on the hearing threshold and frequency selectivity, provide additional evidence for the generation of OAE in the frequency analyzing part of the peripheral auditory system, i.e. in the cochlea.

2.2.6. Evidence against Neural or Middle Ear Origin. A preneural generation of OAE can be evidenced by characteristics that contradict the

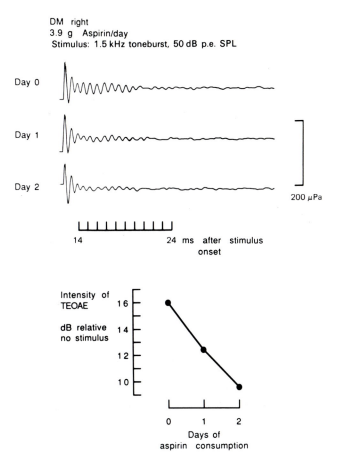

Fig. 1. Influence of aspirin ingestion on short-lasting TEOAE, evoked by a 1.5-kHz toneburst. Upper half: Averaged waveforms on consecutive days. Day 0 represents the day before aspirin ingestion. Lower half: Quantitative changes, computed by spectral densities in the time window 15–20 ms.

typical findings of a neural origin. Such characteristics were demonstrated mainly for TEOAE. They include absence of adaptation with increasing stimulus rates [Kemp, 1978, 1982; Grandori, 1985], complete polarity reversal with stimulus polarity changes [Kemp, 1978; Kemp and Chum, 1980b; Anderson, 1980; Scherer, 1984], and the finding that the TEOAE detection threshold is regularly and clearly lower than the corresponding psychophysical threshold [Kemp, 1978; Wit and Ritsma, 1979; Wilson, 1980b; Zwicker, 1981a, 1983b; Johnsen and Elberling, 1982a, b; Probst et al., 1986; Bonfils et al., 1988a].

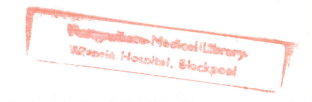

An origin of OAE in the structure of the middle ear could be ruled out by several experimental findings. The middle ear muscles could not be responsible for OAE, which show a main frequency renge of 0.5–6 kHz. Moreover, administration of tubocurarin did not change a SOAE in a guinea pig [Evans et al., 1981], and no systematic changes of SOAE could be detected in human subjects under general anesthesia employing muscle relaxants [Probst and Beck, 1987]. Additionally, other characteristics of OAE, such as long latencies, frequency dispersion, and saturation in the middle intensity range, cannot be explained by known mechanics of the middle ear system. Therefore, a mechanical, energy-dependent process within the cochlea is the most likely generation site of OAE.

2.3. The Middle Ear Factor

Before OAE can be recorded in the ear canal, the vibratory energy has to be conducted in a retrograde fashion from the cochlea through the ossicular chain to the tympanic membrane where it is transduced to acoustic signals. The tympanic membrane functions similar to a loud-speaker membrane. The construction of the middle ear allows such a reverse transmission, though it may be less efficient according to calculations by Kemp [1980, 1981] and Kemp et al. [1986]. Based on the middle ear model of Zwislocki [1962], Kemp [1980] calculated a 12-dB loss for a retrograde transmission at the best frequency range of 1–1.5 kHz. The loss increases at a rate of about 12 dB per octave for lower or higher frequencies. A similar frequency dependence of the transfer function was measured by Schloth [1982], who used tonal suppression of SOAE. The shape of the suppression curves were the same for SOAE of different frequencies. However, the absolute levels of the suppression tones were clearly higher in high-frequency SOAE compared to those around 1 kHz. The findings that SOAE and TEOAE are most readily demonstrated in the frequency range between 1 and 2 kHz may be partially explained by the most efficient retrograde middle ear transmission in this frequency range.

Additional poorly understood, individual factors, such as different resonant frequencies of middle ears, may also be important. This seems to be true in experimentally induced changes of the middle ear and may also be true in pathological changes. Pressure changes in the outer ear canal increase the stiffness of the middle ear and generally decrease the amplitudes of OAE, at least in the frequency range predominantly controlled by stiffness (>1 kHz). Such influences of pressure changes on OAE were examined by Kemp [1981], Wilson and Sutton [1981], and Schloth [1982]. Amplitude reductions and slight frequency increases with positive or negative pressures applied to the outer ear canal were the findings of these studies, pointing to an induced change of the middle ear resonance and possibly of the cochlea as well. Similar changes could be demonstrated during a contralaterally induced stapedial muscle contraction [Schloth, 1982; Schloth and Zwicker, 1983].

Pathological changes of the middle ear transfer function may change the frequency of SOAE and hinder the release of energy from the cochlea. These changes may also sufficiently alter the perception of SOAE so as to induce tinnitus. Some forms of tinnitus in otosclerosis or middle ear effusions may be produced by such mechanisms. However, in most cases, the emission would probably not be recordable in the ear canal, since the very reason for tinnitus would be the lack of an effective retrograde transmission. We examined a case with some audiometric evidence of middle ear disturbance [Probst et al., 1987] in which the rare instances of a still recordable SOAE and a tinnitus matching psychoacoustically to the frequency of this SOAE were present. However, definite proof of this mechanism of tinnitus induction is lacking.

The different recording conditions of the four classes of OAE may also influence the retrograde middle ear transfer. While SOAE represent a steady-state retrograde transmission without interference with external stimuli, there is always a simultaneous anterograde transmission of one or more stimuli when SFOAE and DPOAE are recorded. In TEOAE, the interference between the stimulus and the emission depends on the duration of the impulse stimulus and the latency of the particular TEOAE component. Such interactions between antero- and retrograde transmissions may lead to complex changes of amplitudes and phases of OAE [Matthews, 1983; Matthews and Molnar, 1986].

2.4. Acoustic Probes

By definition, OAE are acoustic energy within the ear canal. Thus, the central element of a system measuring OAE is an acoustic probe incorporating a sensitive microphone. In most cases, the probe is coupled to the ear canal and a possibility to present acoustic stimuli is built in.

The sensitivity and the noise floor of the microphone are of critical importance for the quality of an OAE-measuring system, since the vast majority of OAE are of low-intensity levels. The sensitivity of a microphone is determined by its design and several physical parameters [Wilson, 1980a; Schloth, 1982], such as surface and mass of the microphone membrane or voltage in condenser microphones. Generally, larger microphones are of better quality, providing better sensitivity and less noise floor.

Since commercial probes have only recently become available, most experimental work on OAE was done with custom-built probes of different designs. However, commercial microphones were incorporated in nearly all probes. The most widely, if not exclusively, used kind of microphone was of the condenser type. Two different approaches of applying the micro-phone can be recognized. The more popular approach employs a single or several small microphones, which are placed as close to the ear canal as possible. Figure 2a shows an example of a probe designed with such an approach. Other probes contain more than one subminiature microphone, allowing a reduction of the noise floor by connecting the microphone outputs.

Advantages of such probes include low price, small measuring volume, and small physical dimensions leading to easy handling and relative free-dom from artificial noise introduced through minor movements. Disadvan-tages include lower sensitivity and a higher noise floor when compared to larger microphones with higher quality.

The second approach of probe design consists of a high quality microphone coupled to the ear canal by a connecting tube. Figure 2b depicts such a probe. The main advantages of this type are higher sensi-tivity and a lower noise floor. Since high-quality microphones have typi-cally larger physical dimensions, the connection to the ear canal will be longer and an external supporting system is often necessary. If laboratory animals are examined while under general anesthesia, insignificant amounts of friction-noises are produced and these probes may be advan-tageous. However, such friction-noise is nearly always unavoidable in awake human subjects and the advantages of better sensitivity and lower noise floor may be lost. Additionally, these microphones are usually expensive.

3. Spontaneous Otoacoustic Emissions

SOAE are the only class of OAE not recorded in connection with acoustic stimulation. They are narrowband acoustic signals generated in the cochlea which can be recorded in the ear canal without intentional, external stimulation. It has been shown [Bialek and Wit, 1984] that at least some SOAE are pure tones. As a rule, these emissions are present with relatively minor frequency changes over long time periods of months or years. However, the amplitude of SOAE can vary substantially.

The presence of SOAE was theoretically predicted by Gold in 1948. Case reports of 'objective tinnitus', probably a special form of SOAE, were mentioned sporadically in clinical literature since 1962 [Loebell, 1962]. The first spectral analysis of a SOAE was probably reported by Kumpf and Hocke [1970]. However, Kemp [1979a] can be credited with the initial discovery of SOAE in clinically normal ears. Zurek [1981] was the first to report a larger series of SOAE.

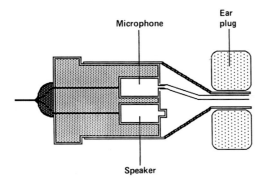

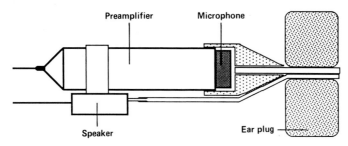

Fig. 2. a Example of a probe design incorporating a small electret microphone (Knowles BT-1751) and a small transducer (Knowles BT-1885). *b* Example of a probe design incorporating a high-quality microphone (B&K 4166) and associated preamplifier (B&K 2619) of relatively large dimensions. Acoustic stimulation is provided through a miniature transducer (Knowles C1-1764).

3.1. Methods of Recording

Since no acoustic stimulation is needed for recording SOAE, an acoustic probe containing just a microphone is sufficient. Besides good sensitivity and a low noise floor of the microphone, the smallest possible measuring volume is advantageous, since the sound pressure of the SOAE will be higher making them more easily recordable. The coupling of the microphone to the ear canal contributes to this aim.

The acoustic background noise in the ear canal is dominated by low-frequency body noises. Noises of blood flow, breathing, muscle contractions, and mandibular joint movements are responsible for the relatively high intrinsic noise floor in the frequency region under 400 Hz. High-pass filters with cutoffs around this frequency are often applied to the microphone signal. Further processing consists in a frequency analysis, generally in the form of 'fast-Fourier transforms' (FFT). Averaging of FFT allows for both a reduction in the amplitudes of random peaks and the employment of an artifact rejection system. However, in contrast to time averaging, it dose not lower the actual noise floor of the recording system itself. Therefore, only a few, usually around 10, averages are sufficient.

The noise floor of the recording, and thereby the 'threshold' of detectable SOAE, are mainly determined by the frequency resolution of the analysis. However, a lower bandwidth usually means analyzing a longer time segment with a greater chance of having some artificial noise in it. Therefore, a compromise has to be chosen and a bandwidth of a few Hertz generally works well. Such artificial interference noise in longer time segments is also often a problem using other methods of frequency analysis, such as narrowband analog or heterodyne filtering.

3.2. Findings in Normal Human Subjects

3.2.1. Incidence. SOAE can be detected in about a third of normal human ears. Table 4 summarizes the findings of ten studies. The results of Fritze [1983a, b], who found 19% SOAE in 37 ears, and Cianfrone and Mattia [1986], who found 26% in 104 ears, were not considered, since these authors used open microphone systems without a coupling to the ear canal. Such systems have different acoustical properties and less sensitivity [Kemp et al., 1986], and the results may not be comparable to those of closed systems. Nearly 1,000 ears were studied and 34% of them, or 43% of subjects, demonstrated one or more SOAE. Thirteen percent of all ears, or 38% of ears with SOAE, showed more than one SOAE per ear. Therefore, multiple SOAE from a single ear are not infrequent, and 10 or more SOAE could be detected in a single ear [Schloth, 1983; Bright and Glattke, 1984].

It seems reasonable to assume that the incidence of SOAE depends on the sensitivity of the recording system. This probably holds true for measuring systems with noise floors above 0 dB SPL. However, a detailed analysis of the ten papers summarized in table 4 does not unequivocally support this assumption. On the one hand, Schloth [1983] and Dallmayr [1985] used very sensitive systems and were able to detect SOAE with levels of -25 dB SPL. These authors felt that they found an increasing incidence of SOAE with a decreasing noise floor. Additionally, multiple SOAE in single ears were mainly found in studies detecting a relatively high overall percentage of SOAE. This overall percentage correlated significantly with the number of ears with multiple SOAE ($r = 0.933$; d.f. $= 7$; $p < 0.001$). These findings seem to support the above-mentioned assumption.

On the other hand, however, it is remarkable that Schloth [1983] detected a similar percentage of SOAE, using a highly sensitive system, as did other investigators, e.g. Zurek [1981], Bright and Glattke [1984], or Wier et al. [1984], using much less sensitive equipment. As a matter of fact, no significant correlations were found between the reported noise floor at

Table 4. Incidence of SOAE in normal ears

	Number of ears examined	Number of ears with SOAE	Percent of ears with SOAE	Number of subjects examined on both ears	Number of subjects with SOAE	Percent of subjects with SOAE	Number of subjects with SOAE in both ears	Percent of subjects with SOAE in both ears
Zurek [1981]	62	21	34	31	15	48	6	19
Tyler and Conrad-Armes [1982]	40	5	13	20	5	25	0	0
Schloth [1983]	128	43	34	64	30	47	13	20
Hammel [1983]	100	25	25	50	17	34	8	16
Bright and Glattke [1984]	144	53	37	72	31	43	22	31
Wier et al. [1984]	92	25	27	45	16	36	7	16
Rabinowitz and Widin [1984]	19	8	42	7	2	29	1	14
Dallmayr [1985]	233	103	44	114	63	55	35	31
Strickland et al. [1985]	138	41	30	67	24	36	13	19
Probst et al. [1986]	28	12	43	14	7	50	5	36
Total	984	336	34.1	484	210	43.4	110	22.7

about 1 kHz of the measuring systems and the incidence of SOAE in the papers described in table 4 (n = 8; r = −0.309) or between this incidence and the level of the weakest SOAE measured, which can be regarded as an indirect indicator of the measuring noise floor (n = 10; r = −0.0512). Additionally, the results of more recently published surveys also vary considerably, though presumably sensitive equipment was generally used. Rebillard et al. [1987] found SOAE in only 19% of 160 ears, Frick and Matthies [1988] in 26% of 62 ears, and Fritze [1988] reported a percentage of 66% SOAE in normal ears. Therefore, no definitive answer can be given to the question whether the incidence of SOAE increases below noise floors of −5 to −10 dB SPL. If this should be the case, the true incidence of SOAE would not be known. Otherwise, about a third of normal human cochleas produce spontaneous oscillations with sufficient amplitudes to be detected in the ear canal as sounds.

If one ear of a subject shows SOAE, the other ear is about twice as likely to also exhibit such emissions as would be expected by chance alone. The pertinent findings supporting this conclusion are summarized in table 4. Both ears were examined in nearly 500 subjects and SOAE were detected in 33% of these ears. A random distribution of SOAE among these ears would result in 11% of binaural SOAE (probability right × probability left; $0.33 \times 0.33 = 0.109$). Actually, 110 subjects or 23% had SOAE in both ears. The difference between this percentage of 23% and the expected percentage of 11% is highly significant ($z = 5.04$; $p < 0.001$). This finding supports the importance of a probable innate and symmetrical cochlear structural feature linked to the generation of SOAE.

3.2.2. Gender and Age Differences. Women seem to exhibit SOAE more often than men. The results of papers reporting the gender differences are summarized in table 5. Overall, SOAE could be found about twice as often in women as in men, a highly significant difference ($z = 3.11$).

The cause of this difference is not clear. A reduction of the incidence of SOAE in men through more occupational or recreational noise exposure is unlikely, since Strickland et al. [1985] found similar differences in infants and children. A possible, but highly speculative explanation would be the smaller physical dimensions of the cochlea in women causing more irregular hair cell patterns. Presumably, such irregularities may be linked to the generation of SOAE [Lonsbury-Martin et al., 1988b].

Based on the results of the study of Strickland et al. [1985], no age-related changes of the incidence of SOAE could be demonstrated. Infants had a somewhat lower incidence [Strickland et al., 1985; Bargones and Burns, 1988]. The recording conditions, however, were less favourable. Additionally, Rebillard et al. [1987] found similar percentages of SOAE in

Table 5. Gender differences of SOAE incidence

	Men (%)	Women (%)
Zurek [1981]	2/10 (20)	12/21 (57)
Hammel [1983]	7/25 (28)	10/25 (40)
Strickland et al. [1985] (children)	6/25 (24)	13/25 (52)
Strickland et al. [1985] (infants)	2/8 (25)	6/13 (46)
Probst et al. [1986]	3/7 (43)	4/7 (57)
Total	20/75 (27)	45/91 (49)

two age groups, 10–29 and 30–50 years. No SOAE were detected in 10 subjects with an age of over 50 years.

3.2.3. Amplitude. The typical amplitudes of SOAE reported in the papers summarized in table 4 varied between −10 and 20 dB SPL. With the exception of rare, high-level emissions that could often be noticed without a microphone, the amplitude of SOAE does not generally exceed 20 dB SPL. A possible explanation for this finding could be a self-limiting saturation mechanism at higher levels [Zwicker, 1979a, 1986b]. In contrast to the stability of frequency, amplitudes of SOAE showed wide variations, at least in time intervals exceeding a few hours [Schloth, 1983; Dallmayr, 1985]. Dallmayr [1985] measured amplitude fluctuations in an ear with 13 SOAE over several weeks and found a standard deviation of 4 dB corresponding to a spreading factor of six. However, Dallmayr's result may not be representative, since interactions of several SOAE in a single ear may have important effects on the amplitudes of SOAE [Burns et al., 1984b]. Short time variations within an hour were generally less than one standard deviation in a study by Frick and Matthies [1988].

Causes of the relative instability of SOAE amplitudes are not known. Changes of the transfer function of the middle ear through pressure differences could be a partial explanation [Schloth and Zwicker, 1983].

3.2.4. Frequency. The typical frequency range of SOAE lies between 0.5 and 6 kHz. Most, if not all, studies (table 4) [Rebilliard et al., 1987; Frick and Matthies, 1988] reported the highest frequency-related incidence of SOAE between 1 and 2 kHz for adult ears. Therefore, this peak incidence seems independent of the frequency responses of the different probes. A possible explanation may be the retrograde transfer function of the middle ear, being most effective in this frequency range, according to

calculations by Kemp [1980]. However, SOAE are common in higher
frequency ranges and emissions up to 9 kHz have been reported [Rebillard
et al., 1987]. Additionally, SOAE of infants appeared to occur in higher
average frequency ranges of 2–7 kHz than in adults [Strickland et al., 1985;
Bargones and Burns, 1988]. A developmental change in SOAE frequencies
seems possible, but not yet experimentally proven. Such changes could
indicate mechanical development of the cochlea, the middle ear, or both
structures.

In contrast to the important fluctuations in amplitude, the frequency
of SOAE shows a remarkable constancy. Values for frequency fluctuations
obtained with repeated measurements over time periods of several months
are summarized in table 6. Köhler et al. [1986] examined eight ears of four
subjects. Seven of these ears showed frequency fluctuations of about 0.4%
as indicated in table 6, but the frequency of a SOAE in one ear changed
nearly 3%. In view of the results of the other studies listed in table 6, such
a large fluctuation has to be considered as exceptional. A clear relationship
between the absolute amount of frequency change and the frequency of the
SOAE was demonstrated by Strickland et al. [1984] and Dallmayr [1985].
Dallmayr [1985] calculated the mean frequency changes to correspond to a
distance of about 2.5 hair cells along the cochlear partition.

Köhler et al. [1986] also compared the frequency changes of the left
and right ear and found significant correlations in two subjects. Therefore,
a systemic influence on frequency changes may be present.

Values of frequency changes for short time periods of minutes to hours
were found to be similar to those of long time periods [Fritze and Köhler,
1985, 1986; Frick and Matthies, 1988]. The finding of frequency stability
indicates that SOAE seem to be generated at specific places on the basilar
membrane and that some structural feature is most likely involved.

3.2.5. Relations between Spontaneous Emissions. Several emissions are
commonly present in ears with SOAE. These multiple emissions may
interact in specific ways, including mutual suppression and generation of
distortion products.

The frequency distance between two emissions seems to be no less than
50 Hz [Schloth, 1983; Dallmayr, 1985] and it is probably related to the
frequency range of SOAE. Schloth [1983] most often found a frequency
difference of 100 Hz, while Dallmayr [1985] reported 0.1 octave or
0.4 Bark. Emissions within less than 50 Hz may be found when FFT
averaging is used. Such emissions were shown to be a single SOAE with
two different and rapidly changing frequency states [Köhler et al., 1986].
Alternatively, there may be a rapid change of mutual suppression between
two SOAE with very similar frequencies. Mutual supressions of SOAE with

Table 6. Frequency changes of SOAE over long time periods

	Frequency changes, %
Schloth [1982]	±1
Fritze [1983a]	±0.4
Bright and Glattke [1984]	±1
Strickland et al. [1984]	±0.1–1
Dallmayr [1985]	±0.4
Köhler et al. [1986]	±0.4
Wilson [1986a]	±0.4–0.8

larger frequency differences were convincingly demonstrated by Burns et al. [1984b] and Champlin and Norton [1987]. Burns et al. [1984b] found another peculiar suppression or activation phenomenon in ears with many SOAE. Two different 'sets' of SOAE were alternatively present and changes from one set to another could be induced by acoustic stimulations. Additionally, SOAE were shown to be generated as distortion products of two other SOAE [Burns et al., 1984b; Jones et al., 1986; Frick and Matthies, 1988].

These interactions among SOAE are probably related to the inherent nonlinear behavior of these emissions. However, the mechanisms involved are poorly understood.

3.2.6. External Influences. The behavior of SOAE may be influenced by external acoustic stimuli, temperature changes, or drugs. The effects of acoustic stimulations include frequency-locking, phase-synchronization, suppression, and fatigue.

Frequency locking of SOAE could be demonstrated within narrow frequency ranges only [Wilson and Sutton, 1981; Zwicker and Schloth, 1984; Rabinowitz and Widin, 1984]. The amount of frequency changes during locking is similar to the spontaneous changes, again indicating the dependency of SOAE on fixed places of the basilar membrane.

The phase of SOAE can be synchronized by acoustic stimuli containing spectral energy at the SOAE frequency [Wilson, 1980a; Wilson and Sutton, 1981]. The duration of synchronizations generally exceeds the duration of the stimulus. This duration depends on the intensity and the time interval between two consecutive stimuli [Schloth, 1982]. The synchronizations were more complete and of longer post-stimulus duration with increasing intensity of the stimulus [Wilson, 1980a; Wit et al., 1981; Schloth, 1982]. However, minimal acoustic energies on the order of only 1 eV were sufficient to induce phase-locking of a SOAE [Wit and Ritsma 1983a, b].

Spontaneous emissions are ideal means for the study of suppression contours and many investigators reported such experiments (table 3). While the typical SOAE suppression tuning curve is similar to the well-known psychophysical tuning curve, the following characteristics can be summarized from experimental findings (table 3): (1) Most effective suppression was obtained at a frequency slightly higher than the SOAE frequency [Wilson, 1980a; Wilson and Sutton, 1981; Zurek, 1981; Schloth, 1982; Ruggero et al., 1983; Dallmayr, 1985; Rebillard et al., 1987; Bargones and Burns, 1988]. (2) The degree of suppression increased more rapidly when suppression tones with lower frequencies than the SOAE were used compared to tones with higher frequencies [Zurek, 1981; Schloth, 1982; Rabinowitz and Widin, 1984]. (3) The high frequency suppression contour was often found not to be monotonous showing additional minima [Zurek, 1981; Dallmayr, 1985; Bargones and Burns, 1988].

This nonmonotonous behavior of SOAE suppression curves was thought to be related to the level of SOAE by Zwicker [1986b], based on results obtained in a hardware cochlear model. However, experimental findings in humans do not support this suggestion. While Zurek [1981] found additional minima in relatively loud SOAE of 9 dB SPL, Dallmayr demonstrated them in emissions of only −10 dB SPL. Additionally, other investigators [Wilson and Sutton, 1981; Schloth, 1982; Rabinowitz and Widin, 1984; Bargones and Burns, 1988] found no minima examining emissions with levels of 10–20 dB SPL.

The temporal course of suppression depends on the intensity of the external tone. After a tone of short duration that induced a complete suppression, the SOAE reappeared with a time delay of about 5.5 ms [Schloth and Zwicker, 1983; Dallmayr, 1985]. Thereafter, the amplitude increased exponentially to its original value with a time constant between 13 ms [Schloth and Zwicker, 1983] and 23 ms [Dallmayr, 1985]. More intense stimuli can induce fatigue of SOAE with time courses similar to the well-known psychoacoustical temporary threshold shifts. However, the exact amplitude and frequency changes were found to be complex and individually different [Kemp, 1981, 1986, 1988; Norton et al., 1987; Champlin and Norton, 1987]. Slow oscillatory recovery functions with overshooting were found by Kemp [1981, 1986, 1988] after low-frequency fatiguing exposures. He related these changes to slow acting cochlear control mechanisms. Fatiguing could be demonstrated with stimuli as low as 100 dB for less than 30 s [Norton et al., 1987].

The influence of contralateral stimulation on SOAE is equivocal. While most investigators [Schloth and Zwicker, 1983; Grose, 1983; Rabinowitz and Widin, 1984] only found effects that could be explained by the stapedial reflex or crossed stimulations, Mott et al. [1987] thought they demonstrated effects independent of these factors.

Aspirin, taken in doses of about 4 g per day, reduced or abolished the amplitudes of SOAE in normal subjects [McFadden and Plattsmier, 1984; Long et al., 1986; Wier et al., 1988].

General anesthesia induced unsystematical amplitude and frequency changes of SOAE [Probst and Beck, 1987; Beck and Probst, 1988]. Two examples of the time courses of such changes are shown in figure 3.

Generally, SOAE were not abolished during anesthesia. Systematic patterns of changes could not be recognized. A minority of the examined SOAE showed negatively correlated changes of amplitudes and frequencies indicating a possible middle ear influence through the use of nitrous oxide and muscle relaxants.

A diurnal influence upon the frequency of SOAE was found by Wit [1985]. The average frequency reduction from morning to evening amounted to 3 Hz. An influence of the body temperature was considered as a possible explanation. However, Wilson [1986a] could not demonstrate such an influence examining menstrual cycles, diurnal patterns, and experimentally induced temperature changes by ear irrigations.

3.3. Findings in Patients

SOAE can also be detected in ears with hearing loss, though probably less frequently and only in frequency ranges with normal or nearly normal hearing. Possible exceptions are loud SOAE that can be heard form rare subjects, even without a microphone.

3.3.1. High-Level Emissions. Objective, tonal sounds from ears have been recognized for many years in clinical literature. Table 7 summarizes the findings of papers reporting such sounds, most of which were published before the discovery of SOAE by Kemp [1979a]. These sounds were exceptional in their tonal, high-frequency character not consistent with an origin from blood vessels or muscles. Nevertheless, they were generally termed 'objective tinnitus'. However, since most subjects were unaware of their emitted sounds and tinnitus is defined as a subjective sensation [Tinnitus, 1981], this term is not correct. To distinguish this exceptional form of SOAE from the commonly found variety, the term 'high-level SOAE' will be applied.

The following conclusions can be drawn from table 7: (1) These high-level SOAE were often detected in children who emitted sounds of high intensities. (2) No gender differences were apparent. (3) High-level SOAE were often present binaurally. (4) Their frequencies were clearly higher than those of SOAE found in surveys of normal subjects.

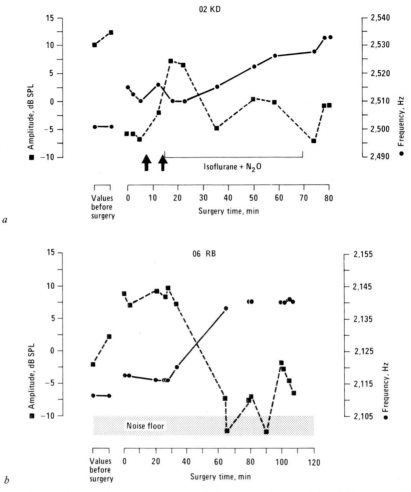

Fig. 3. Graphs of changes of amplitude (squares, left ordinate) and frequency (dots, right ordinate) of SOAE during general anesthesia. Left arrow: Induction of anesthesia. Second arrow: Intubation. *a* Unsystematic and uncorrelated changes of amplitude and frequency. *b* Changes with a significant inverse correlation ($r = -0.82$, $p < 0.001$).

In about half of the cases [Loebell, 1962; Kumpf and Hoke, 1970; Glanville et al., 1971] listed in table 7, general anesthesia with muscle relaxants was applied in order to test for a muscular generation of these unusual sounds. No major changes of the sound were reported. Hearing loss of the involved ear in the frequency range of the high-level SOAE was reported by Glanville et al. [1971], Huizing and Spoor [1973], and Yamamoto et al. [1987].

Table 7. Findings in subjects with high-level SOAE

	Age years	Gender	Side	Number of SOAE	Ampl. dB SPL	Freq. kHz
Loebell [1962]	3	M	r	1	>30	≈5
			l	1	>40	≈5.5
Citron [1969]	4	F	r	1	>30	7.5–8
			l	1	>30	7.5–8
Kumpf and Hoke [1970]		F	r	1	15 to 20	4.2
Glanville et al. [1971]	26	M	l	3	−1 to 20	5.95–6.51
	4	M	r	11	1 to 35	6.31–10.83
			l	9	−4 to 38	5.64–14.14
	0.3	F	r	10	−2 to 21	7.55–9.39
			l	11	14 to 24	7.07–13.24
Huizing and Spoor [1973]	22	F	r	1	35	3.4
Yamamoto et al. [1987]	25	M	r	1	37	6.1

Kumpf and Hoke [1970] tested a woman probably suffering from Ménière's disease on the left side. No emissions were detected on this side. However, a tone of 15–20 dB was found on the right side 'with a sensitive microphone', which could not be heard by the unaided ear. A relationship to the left-sided ear disease could not be established. Therefore, this report probably contained the first description of a 'true' SOAE. The meaning of this finding was not recognized at that time.

Glanville et al. [1971] reported on a family emitting sounds. The father and two children exhibited high-level SOAE. Congenital deafness was known on the father's side of the family. The children, a boy and a girl, were reexamined by Wilson and Sutton [1983] 13 years later. The boy showed 19 SOAE on the right and 5 emissions on the left side in the frequency range between 2.8 and 12 kHz. Even more emissions were found in the girl's ears, namely 18 on the right and 23 on the left side; their frequencies ranged from 1.4 to 17 kHz. All emissions with amplitudes greater than 20 dB SPL had frequencies above 5 kHz. The audiograms of three of the four ears showed high frequency dips at about 8 kHz, and the hearing loss of the boy was unchanged compared with the examination 13 years earlier. The high-level SOAE at high frequencies could not be synchronized by click stimuli and, additionally, the slopes of tuning curves of these emissions were less steep than generally found in 'normal' SOAE.

Another family with several members demonstrating SOAE with levels of 40 dB and with high frequencies was mentioned by Strickland et al. [1984]. However, no further details were described.

The findings of these case reports indicate that these 'high-level' SOAE are probably a special form of SOAE. Such high-level SOAE seem to be rare, and they do not follow the same behavior as other SOAE. In particular, their amplitudes exceed 20 dB and may not show the assumed amplitude limitations of other SOAE. Moreover, they do not synchronize to short stimuli, and a relationship to pathological changes of the cochlea seems to exist with a possible genetic background.

3.3.2. Ears with Hearing Loss. There is general agreement that SOAE can be present in ears with important hearing loss. Zurek [1981] reported in his first series of SOAE about an ear with SOAE and a high-frequency hearing loss and, later, Tyler and Conrad-Armes [1982] described a similar case. Additional ears with a coexistence of hearing loss and SOAE were reported by Fritze [1983a, b], Bright and Glattke [1984], Probst et al. [1987], Penner and Burns [1987], and Rebillard et al. [1987].

The hearing threshold at the frequency of SOAE and the relationship between the incidence of SOAE and hearing loss appear less clear in these reports. However, hearing losses at SOAE frequencies above 30 dB HL were only reported for high-level SOAE as described above. Fritze [1983a, b] was the only investigator reporting a significantly higher incidence of SOAE in patients with 'moderate' hearing loss (7 of 12 ears, 58%) compared to normal hearing subjects (7 of 37 ears, 19%, $\chi^2 = 6.9$, p < 0.01). Lower incidences in ears with mild sensorineural losses than in normal ears were found by Bright and Glattke [1984] (32 versus 43%), and Probst et al. [1987] (22 versus 43%). Penner and Burns [1987] reported a percentage of 17% SOAE in such ears, and Rebillard et al. [1987] found similar incidences of SOAE in normals (25%) and in patients with hearing loss (23%). In normals, the hearing threshold at the SOAE frequency tended to be more sensitive than at adjacent frequencies [Schloth, 1982, 1983; Ruggero et al., 1983; Zwicker and Schloth, 1984; Burns et al., 1984a; Long et al., 1986]. Direct measurements of the hearing thresholds at the SOAE frequency in patients are not available. However, such thresholds were estimated from interpolations between the standard audiometric frequencies and showed an average hearing loss of 9 dB HL, never exceeding 15 dB HL [Probst et al., 1987]. This finding indicated an essentially normal threshold at SOAE frequencies in ears with hearing losses.

The etiology causing the hearing loss may influence the incidence of SOAE in ears with high frequency hearing loss. Ears with presumably noise induced hearing loss showed significantly less SOAE than ears with similar hearing loss due to other etiological factors [Probst et al., 1987]. However, in anecdotal case reports [Flottorp, 1953; Wilson and Sutton, 1981; Norton and Mott, 1987; Rebillard et al., 1987], the appearance of SOAE was linked to acute acoustic injuries of the cochlea. In conclusion, it remains unclear if SOAE are associated with variations of the normal cochlea and/or subtle pathological changes.

3.3.3. Tinnitus and Spontaneous Emissions. The initial hope [Wilson and Sutton, 1981] that SOAE may be an objective correlate to subjective tinnitus quickly faded. McFadden and Wightman [1983] reviewed the literature and came to the conclusion 'that spontaneous acoustic emissions are commonly observed objectively, but only infrequently observed subjectively'. Since then, additional studies have supported this statement [Hazell, 1984; Wilson, 1986b; Probst et al., 1987; Penner and Burns, 1987; Rebillard et al., 1987]. Particularly convincing evidence against an association between tinnitus and SOAE was presented by Penner and Burns [1987]. These investigators demonstrated that independent masking of either tinnitus or SOAE was possible without influencing SOAE or tinnitus, respectively.

3.4. Findings in Animals

The incidence of SOAE in animals depends on the species. Table 8 summarizes the findings of reported SOAE from animals. About half of the reports listed in table 8 described emissions which were detected by chance and not in systematic surveys [Evans et al., 1981; Decker and Fritsch, 1982; Rabinowitz and Widin, 1984; Ruggero et al., 1984]. These emissions resemble the high-level SOAE of human ears in their frequencies, high amplitudes and sporadic appearance. Evans et al. [1981] reported synchronizations similar to those commonly found in humans, but with qualitative differences in the suppression tuning curve. Broad tuning was also measured by Ruggero et al. [1984], who found a probable hearing loss in the frequency range of the emission.

Systematic surveys discovered SOAE rarely or not at all in most common laboratory animals. It can be concluded from several papers that unsuccessful surveys for SOAE were carried out in guinea pigs [Wit and Ritsma, 1980; Zwicker and Manley, 1981], cats [Wilson, 1980c], caimans [Strack, 1986], gerbils [Schmiedt and Adams, 1981], starlings [Manley et al., 1987], and rabbits [Lonsbury-Martin et al., 1987], though formal data were generally not provided by these papers. Surveys detecting SOAE were reported for frogs [Palmer and Wilson, 1982, bilateral SOAE in 7 of 12 animals], bats [Kössl and Vater, 1985, 1 of 30 ears], chinchillas [Zurek and Clark, 1981] and primates [Martin et al., 1985; Lonsbury-Martin and Martin, 1988].

3.4.1. Chinchillas. The findings in chinchillas [Zurek and Clark, 1981; Clark et al., 1984] are particularly interesting in regard to a possible

Table 8. SOAE reported in animals (s. = side)

	Species	Number of animals	Freq. kHz	Ampl. dB SPL
Evans et al. [1981]	guinea pig	1 one s.	1.16	21
Zurek and Clark [1981]	chinchilla	2 one s.	≈4.65/5.75 ≈6.5	35/15 25
Palmer and Wilson [1982]	frog	7 both s.	≈1–2	−10 to 0
Decker and Fritsch [1982]	dog	1 one s.	10.28	15
Ruggero et al. [1984]	dog	1 both s.	9.1 9.5–11.5	59 20 to 50
Rabinowitz and Widin [1984]	dog	1 one s.	≈5	50
Kössl and Vater [1985]	bat	1 one s.	63.5	40
Martin et al. [1985]	primate	3 one s.	2.2–3.91 1.43/1.57 3.66–4.91	2 to 10 15/3 2 to 7
Lonsbury-Martin and Martin [1988]	macaque	3 both s. 6 one s.	1.4–8	−13 to 10

explanation of SOAE-generating mechanisms. No SOAE was detected in 26 ears of 17 animals not exposed to noise. However, two of 17 animals exhibited SOAE after damaging noise exposure. Eleven chinchillas were examined before and after noise exposure; only one ear had an SOAE after the exposure. Six animals were tested only after exposure and one of those ears showed an additional SOAE. Thus, it appears that SOAE could be induced by noise exposure under specific circumstances. These SOAE resembled 'high-level SOAE' in some characteristics. They were relatively loud and had high frequencies (table 8). Suppression tuning curves had similar shapes as those found in humans, but growth of suppression was somewhat different. In contrast to the findings in humans, suppression increased at about the same rate with stimuli of higher and lower frequencies.

The two ears with SOAE were examined histologically, along with 18 other ears exposed to similar noise intensities. Circumscribed cochlear lesions with destruction of the organ of Corti were found in the region corresponding roughly to the emitted frequency. However, similar defects were found in 13 of the 18 other ears. Therefore, a specific pathohistological substrate could not be found, but SOAE were presumably generated in the vicinity of cochlear lesions.

3.4.2. Primates. Nonhuman primates, especially macaque monkeys, seem to have more readily detectable SOAE than other species [Martin et al., 1985; Lonsbury-Martin and Martin, 1988]. Moreover, frequency and amplitude ranges of their SOAE are similar to those found in humans. In two surveys, macaque monkeys were found to have SOAE in 7 and 9% [Martin et al., 1985; Lonsbury-Martin and Martin, 1988]. A total of 34 SOAE was detected in 15 ears of 143 animals. Thus, multiple emissions per ear were the rule and only three ears emitted a single SOAE. Ten monkeys were females and two males, reflecting the typical gender distribution within breeding colonies. Though the overall incidence of SOAE is clearly lower in macaque monkeys than in humans, the characteristics of the SOAE are quite similar. A detailed study of OAE in one of the monkeys from the above-mentioned surveys furnished further evidence for this similarity [Martin et al., 1988], in that frequency and amplitude distributions of SOAE, their bandwidths and suppression tuning curves were not substantially different from those found in human SOAE.

A histological examination [Lonsbury-Martin et al., 1988b] of the two ears of this monkey revealed no significant hair cell loss and no circumscribed lesions similar to those found in chinchillas. However, a general irregularity of the hair cell pattern, more pronounced in the apical than the basal region, was found. This is a common finding in both macaque monkeys [Hawkins et al., 1985; Lonsbury-Martin et al., 1988b] and humans [Engström et al., 1966; Bredberg, 1968]. A fourth row of outer hair cells was inconsistently present. Figure 4 shows drawings of the hair cell pattern at three different regions along the cochlea of these ears.

These investigations demonstrated that SOAE can occur in ears without obvious pathohistological changes. Further implications of these findings will be discussed later, together with the findings in other OAE. However, differences in the generation of SOAE such as those found in this monkey, and presumably in humans, and those found in chinchillas seem conceivable.

4. Transiently Evoked Otoacoustic Emissions

TEOAE can be recorded in the ear canal following a transient acoustic stimulation, such as a click. They exhibit typical characteristics including nonlinear growth with saturation at moderate levels of stimulation, frequency dispersion, and latency. The pioneering paper of Kemp [1978] described TEOAE for the first time. Since then, many additional investigations have been carried out, and TEOAE are in the process of becoming an accepted means for clinical hearing examination.

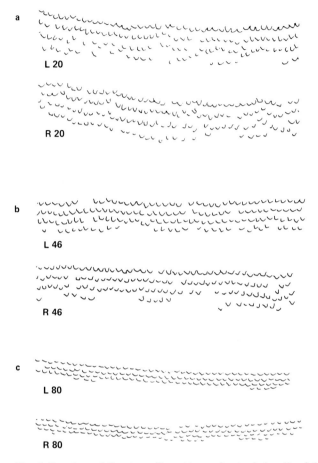

Fig. 4. Drawings of the stereocilia patterns of outer hair cells of the right (R) and left (L) ears of a monkey with SOAE. *a* Apical region. *b* Middle region. *c* Basal region. From Lonsbury-Martin et al. [1988b], with permission of the publisher.

4.1. Methods of Recording

Acoustic probes for the recording of TEOAE need a means for acoustic stimulation, in contrast to the recording technique for SOAE. Ideally, a relatively flat frequency response curve in the range between 0.3 and 8 kHz should be obtained within the ear canal for both the recording microphone and the acoustic stimulus. The probe microphone can be used for monitoring the stimulus level and its acoustic waveform, thereby assuring a good and constant probe fit [Bray and Kemp, 1987].

Commonly used transient stimuli are rectangular or Gaussian-shaped clicks, single sinusoids, half sinusoids, or tonebursts. The quality of the transducer is generally not critical and miniature speakers, such as those used in hearing aids, are adequate. For the recording of TEOAE, the microphone signal is averaged with a time lock to the transient stimulus, usually after high-pass filtering at a frequency of 300–500 Hz. Basically, the same rules apply for this averaging procedure as they do for the recording of evoked auditory responses measuring bioelectrical signals. In the case of TEOAE, the acoustic waveform following the short stimulus is averaged. A design for artifact rejections during averaging is indispensable for practical and clinical purposes. Artifact rejection can be determined by preselected noise levels or by adaptive strategies using subaverages after linear cancellation [Bray and Kemp, 1987].

Such linear cancellation procedures are the most important verifications of TEOAE and essential for practical purposes, since ringing in individual ear canals with probe couplings of different qualities may produce waveforms that are similar to TEOAE. The linear cancellation is based on the nonlinear growth of TEOAE, which shows strong saturations at medium stimulus levels of about 60 dB SPL, in contrast to the linear growth of acoustic ringing [Kemp et al., 1986].

There are at least two different procedures to cancel the linear elements in averaged waveforms. One is using mathematical waveform manipulations, while the other employs special stimulus presentations. Waveform manipulations were generally accomplished off-line. An example of such a manipulation is provided in figure 5.

An average to a stimulus of 70 dB (right ear) or 60 dB (left ear) was recorded first. A second average to a 6-dB louder stimulus, having double the amplitude, was then recorded with half the gain of the previous recording. Thus, linearly growing components would have the same amplitude in both recordings and only nonlinear components are preserved when the two recordings are subtracted from each other. Essentially the same procedure was used in different ways by many investigators [Wit and Kahmann, 1982; Wit and Ritsma, 1983a; Kemp et al., 1986; Probst et al., 1986].

A cancellation of linear waveform components can also be achieved by a special stimulus presentation. Kemp et al. [1986] and Bray and Kemp [1987] used sets of four stimuli, three identical clicks with the same polarity and the same relatively low stimulation level, and a fourth click with opposite polarity and three times the amplitude of the former stimuli. Thus, the stimuli waveform and its ringing are cancelled after each train of four clicks presentation. No off-line manipulations are necessary after such a procedure, and artifact rejection can be adjusted to the subaverages obtained after four clicks. All cancellation procedures lead to a reduction of

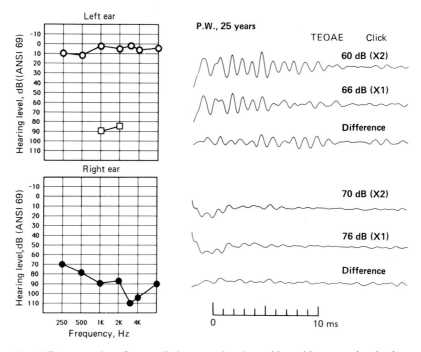

Fig. 5. Demonstration of a cancellation procedure in a subject with a severe hearing loss on the right side due to a mumps infection, along with normal hearing on the left side. Top: The derived waveform shows clear TEOAE after cancellation of linearly growing components. Bottom: Low-frequency dominated ringing after a relatively loud click stimulus, the derived waveform (difference) shows no TEOAE.

TEOAE amplitudes, this reduction being dependent on the degree of TEOAE saturation [Kemp et al., 1986]. However, such a relatively small loss of the amplitude is outweighed by a reliable identification of TEOAE.

A frequency analysis of averaged waveforms, generally in the form of FFT, is necessary for correct interpretations of TEOAE. Alternatively, FFT averages can be taken after each stimulus without previous time averaging [Wit et al., 1981]. Signals showing less synchronization by the short stimulus may be identified more easily with such a procedure, since they could be partially cancelled by time-locked averaging.

To test for reproducibility of two sequentially or simultaneously averaged waveforms, cross-correlations are widely employed [Johnsen and Elberling, 1982a; Elberling et al., 1985; Kemp et al., 1986; Bray and Kemp, 1987; Stevens, 1988]. Such a correlation can be very helpful, but only after linear cancellations, since ringing of the stimulus itself is repeatable and can be misleading in the original waveform.

4.2. Findings in Normal Human Subjects

4.2.1. Incidence in Adults. Transiently evoked emissions can be detected in nearly all human ears with normal hearing, regardless of age or gender. Table 9 summarizes results reported in the literature.

Excluding the results of van Dijk and Wit [1987], TEOAE were found in 98% of ears with normal hearing. Why van Dijk and Wit [1987] obtained a much lower incidence than all other studies is not entirely clear. Indeed, the incidence reported by these investigators is similar to the incidence of SOAE and they may well have only detected synchronized SOAE. Their recording system was a commercially available apparatus for TEOAE measurements (Peters AP 200) and the criterion adopted by van Dijk and Wit, emissions 3 dB above the noise floor and a coefficient of 70% in the cross-correlation of two recordings, seemed reasonable. A flaw in the design of this apparatus must be assumed [Bray and Kemp, 1987], since Kemp et al. [1986] obtained TEOAE in 100% of normal ears using a similar apparatus of much improved design.

Occasional failure to detect TEOAE in ears with normal hearing has to be expected in clinical situations, be it for anatomical reasons of the ear-canal or middle ear, equipment related problems, or noise problems. However, it is unclear if normal ears exist without TEOAE, even when tested carefully with special laboratory equipment. Our investigations [Probst et al., 1986] indicate that the spectrum of the stimulus may be important. Figure 6 shows an example of TEOAE from an ear in which no click-response could be detected. However, tonebursts evoked short, but clear, emissions showing broad spectral peaks at the toneburst frequencies.

Though a maximal amount of information may be obtained by a broadband stimulus under most circumstances [Elberling et al., 1985; Kemp et al., 1986], the response may be difficult to detect in some ears. The reason for this finding could be a very broadly tuned response which is difficult to detect or mutual cancellations of TEOAE components. The linear superposition of the toneburst responses in figure 6, resulting in a similar waveform as the click response, could provide evidence for both mechanisms.

In conclusion, TEOAE can be recorded in the vast majority, if not all, normal hearing ears and TEOAE seem to be a general property of the human peripheral auditory system. Under ordinary conditions, however, the limitations of the stimulus and recording systems, variations of anatomy, and criteria used to define these emissions may all influence the actual incidence of TEOAE.

4.2.2. Age Differences. The literature generally agrees on the finding that TEOAE are detected in similar proportions in infants or children with normal hearing as found in adults [Stevens et al., 1987; Johnsen et al., 1988;

Table 9. Incidence of TEOAE in normal human ears

	Number of tested ears	Number of ears with TEOAE	Percent of ears with TEOAE	Stimulus
Kemp [1978]	35	35	100	click 100 μs
Rutten [1980a]	19	18	95	click 60 μs, TB
Schloth [1982]	34	31	91	single sinus. 1.4 kHz
Johnsen and Elberling [1982a]	20	20	100	half sinus. 2 kHz
Grandori [1983]	23	22	96	click 100 μs
Zwicker [1983a]	30	21	70	single sinus. 1.3 kHz
Horst et al. [1983]	16	12	75	click
Elberling et al. [1985]	199	199	100	single sinus. 2 kHz
Probst et al. [1986]	28	28	100	click 100 μs, TB
Kemp et al. [1986]	150	150	100	click 100 μs
Dijk and Wit [1987]	210	85	40	click 100 μs
Stevens [1988]	36	35	97	click 100 μs
Bonfils et al. [1988a]	262	262	100	click 100 μs
Total	1,062	918	86	
Total without van Dijk and Wit [1987]	852	833	98	

Bonfils et al., 1988c, d]. Amplitudes of TEOAE in infants may be larger than under comparable conditions in adults [Bray and Kemp, 1987].

Bonfils et al. [1988a, d] reported age-related incidences of TEOAE in age groups from less than 10 years to more than 60 years. Transiently evoked emissions were detected in all ears of subjects less than 60 years old. Above this age, the incidence of TEOAE fell to 35%. However, the hearing of this highest age group could be considered normal only in age-adjusted terms, and the average subjective click threshold of this group of subjects was 29 dB HL. Therefore, the drop in TEOAE incidence in the age group over 60 years may have been caused largely by hearing loss and not by age alone.

4.2.3. Duration. The durations of TEOAE show a wide range from a few ms up to several hundreds of ms [Wit and Ritsma, 1980]. On the basis of TEOAE duration, two groups of TEOAE were distinguished [Zwicker, 1983a; Probst et al., 1986]: 'short' and 'long' TEOAE. Zwicker [1983a] did not separate the two groups by a fixed time limit, but he called emissions without amplitude modulations 'short' TEOAE, and those showing such

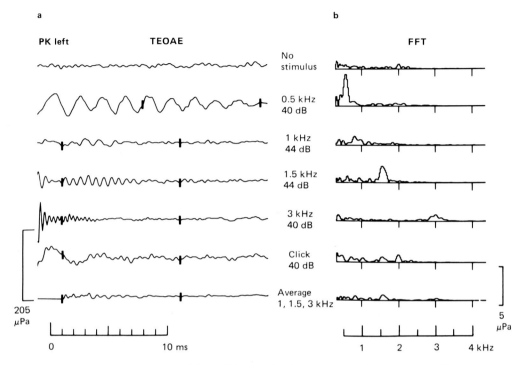

Fig. 6. TEOAE of an ear without click-evoked emissions. *a* time domaine averages for tonebursts and clicks. Click response shows only low frequency ringing along with background noise. Bottom trace represents offline average of responses to 1, 1.5, and 3 kHz, demonstrating linear superposition of TEOAE. *b* Frequency-amplitude spectra of 10 ms time window indicated by vertical bars in *a*. From Probst et al. [1986], with permission of the publisher.

modulations 'long' emissions. However, we [Probst et al., 1986] demonstrated that this criterion may be dependent on the type of stimulus. While clicks or tonebursts of certain frequencies may induce amplitude modulations, a toneburst of another frequency may fail to do so in the same ear. Therefore, we chose an empirical boundary of 20 ms after the click onset to differentiate between long and short TEOAE.

Short TEOAE were found in 18% of normal ears using the limit of 20 ms [Probst et al., 1986]. Schloth [1982] reported a similar percentage of 21% using the criterion of Zwicker [1983a]. None of the ears with short TEOAE showed SOAE. In contrast, SOAE could be detected in about 50% of ears with long TEOAE [Probst et al., 1986]. Frequency dispersion and/or amplitude modulations were evident in the waveforms of these long TEOAE, both phenomena indicating the presence of more than one dominant emission frequency in the response amplitude spectrum. Such dominant emission frequencies may be SOAE synchronized by the transient stimulus and lead regularly to 'long' TEOAE; alternatively, they may be generated by evoked damped oscillations at certain frequency places. Therefore, the duration of TEOAE is intimately related to the spectral content of the frequency response.

Clinically, duration by itself is difficult to measure and only of relative value. The classification of TEOAE based on durations is arbitrary and transitions from one form to another are possible depending on stimulus parameters. However, the fact remains that ears with apparently indistinguishable conventional audiometric findings can exhibit very different TEOAE.

4.2.4. Spectrum. The amplitude spectrum of TEOAE is dominated by several emission frequencies in the majority of ears [Kemp, 1981; Wit et al., 1981; Zwicker and Schloth, 1984; Probst et al., 1986; Bonfils et al., 1988a]. These emission frequencies are evoked when a stimulus contains spectral energy at the specific frequency, independent of stimulus type or intensity. Related to the basilar membrane, these frequencies are emitted by generators with 'fixed' places [Kemp, 1986].

The dominant emission frequencies themselves, their numbers, and their tuning is different for each ear. Spontaneous emissions represent emissions with particular high tuning and, as already mentioned, with long durations. However, additional dominant frequencies, not detectable as SOAE, could be found regularly in the spectrum of TEOAE of ears with SOAE [Wit et al., 1981; Probst et al., 1986]. An example is shown in figure 7.

An average of seven distinct frequencies in the spectrum of the click-evoked emissions were found in ears with SOAE [Probst et al., 1986]. Only an average of two to three of them were detected as SOAE. Moreover, the emission frequencies not corresponding to a SOAE could show similar amplitude and tuning as those represented by SOAE. Emission frequencies with similar properties were also found in ears without SOAE, though the average number was only four per ear. The already mentioned frequency dispersion and amplitude modulation are generated through an interaction of these multiple, fixed emission frequencies.

Such emission frequencies are most often found in the range of 0.5–4 kHz [Wit et al., 1981; Zwicker and Schloth, 1984; Elberling et al., 1985; Probst et al., 1986]. The long-time stability of these frequencies is also similar to those found in SOAE [Kemp, 1978, 1982; Kemp et al., 1986; Wilson, 1980a; Antonelli and Grandori, 1986].

The waveform of TEOAE is dependent on the number and tuning of the 'fixed' emission frequencies and on the spectrum of the stimulus. An

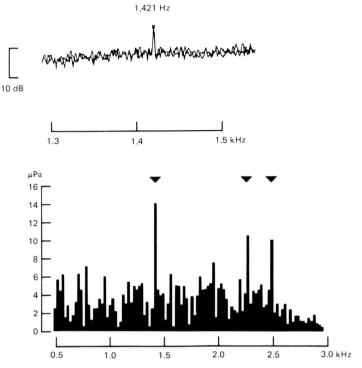

Fig. 7. Spectra in the unstimulated ear canal (top) and after a click stimulation (bottom). Top: Two spectra are replicated, indicating a SOAE at 1,421 Hz. No additional SOAE were detected in this ear in the frequency range between 0.5 and 5 kHz. Noise floor is about −10 dB SPL. Bottom: Spectrum of click-evoked emissions, showing a peak at the frequency corresponding to the SOAE frequency (1,421 Hz), and two additional peaks at 2,261 and 2,480 Hz, representing nonspontaneously emitting frequencies.

example of the effect of different stimuli is shown in figure 8. Tonebursts with relatively narrow spectra may each evoke very different waveforms.

As shown in figure 8, no highly tuned, dominant emission frequency was present in this ear within the spectral energy of the 1-kHz toneburst, leading to a short emission with low amplitude after this stimulus. However, in the same ear, the 1.5-kHz toneburst synchronized a SOAE at about that frequency, leading to a stable waveform of high amplitude. Amplitude modulation is evident at the beginning of this TEOAE, indicating that the 1.5-kHz toneburst evoked other emission frequencies within its spectral energy which oscillated for a shorter time than the synchronized SOAE. Finally, the broad spectrum of the click evoked many emission frequencies with different damping leading to a complex waveform.

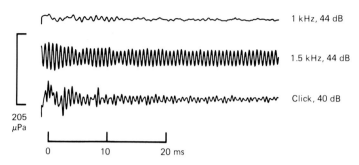

Fig. 8. TEOAE evoked by different stimuli in the same ear. The 1-kHz tone burst evoked a short, low-amplitude emission, the 1.5-kHz tone burst synchronized a SOAE at about this frequency, and the broadband click stimulated many emitting frequencies leading to a complex waveform.

It was shown that emission frequencies generally superimpose linearly [Elberling et al., 1985; Probst et al., 1986]. Complicated, nonlinear interactions, however, such as those found among SOAE, cannot be excluded, especially if emission frequencies are close together.

In a minority of ears, approximately 20% [Schloth, 1982; Probst et al., 1986], dominant, fixed emission frequencies are difficult to demonstrate. An example was shown in figure 6 (page 31). While no TEOAE could be recognized after the click stimulus, tonebursts evoked TEOAE which showed similar spectra as the tonebursts themselves. Indeed, a second spectral component, besides fixed frequencies, seems to be a broadly tuned, continuous frequency band [Probst et al., 1986; Bray and Kemp, 1987; Norton and Neely, 1987; Bonfils et al., 1988a]. As shown in figure 6, this component may be dependent on the spectrum of the stimulus [Probst et al., 1986; Norton and Neely, 1987] and it may be difficult to detect in broadband click-evoked emissions. Bonfils et al. [1988a] found the frequency band of this component to range between 0.5 and 2.5 kHz, decreasing with age and with higher TEOAE thresholds. Maximum amplitudes of this TEOAE component were located between 1 and 2 kHz.

In summary, then, TEOAE are dominated by fixed frequencies of individually different numbers and places in most clinically normal ears. A second, broadly tuned frequency component also seems to be present. While the first component is relatively easy to detect, the second may be difficult to demonstrate. Information at specific, standardized frequencies can be obtained for the second component only. It is still unclear, for the moment, if this is possible.

4.2.5. Latency. Transiently evoked emissions appear in the human ear canal with a certain latency, which is dependent on the frequency of the emission. High frequencies have shorter latencies than low frequencies. Several important difficulties hamper the measurements of latencies, including difficulties in separating the stimulus tail from the beginning of the TEOAE, and determination of the beginning of specific components in a multifrequency event. Additionally, exact latency measurements may not be possible in a complex, multifrequency, nonlinear response such as TEOAE [Anderson, 1980; Norton and Neely, 1987]. For example, the widely used measurements of 'group latencies' [Johnsen and Elberling, 1982b; Norton and Neely, 1985] is a technique developed for linear systems. It measures the point of time when the energy of TEOAE reaches a maximum in relation to frequencies; thus, the actual beginning of a frequency component is not measured.

Table 10 summarizes reported latency values from the literature. The values are approximations, since wide individual variations were reported that may be partly related to the above-mentioned difficulties.

The values of table 10 are substantially longer than those found for latencies of summed action potentials [Eggermont, 1979]. However, the difference can probably be explained by the necessity of additional, retrograde traveling time and the use of much lower stimulus levels than normally used for evoked potentials [Anderson, 1980; Norton and Neely, 1985; Neely et al., 1986, 1988]. If this assumption is true, shorter latencies with higher stimulus levels should be expected. While Johnsen and Elberling [1982a], Schloth [1982], and Wilson [1980c] found essentially unchanged latencies with different stimulus levels, Norton and Neely [1985, 1987] and Johnsen et al. [1988] in a later study demonstrated such an inverse relationship between stimulus level and latency.

Similar to the linear superposition of frequency components, the latencies of TEOAE were shown to superpose in the same way [Zwicker, 1983a]. Each cycle of a stimulating toneburst evoked TEOAE components that added together linearly with constant latencies.

If latency is a useful parameter in clinical TEOAE testing, it remains to be demonstrated. New recording techniques may simplify the measurement of latency, but fundamental difficulties may persist.

4.2.6. Detection Threshold. Detection thresholds of TEOAE are often lower than the corresponding psychoacoustic threshold [Kemp, 1978; Wit and Ritsma, 1979; Wilson, 1980b; Zwicker, 1981a, 1983b; Johnsen and Elberling, 1982a, b; Probst et al., 1986; Bonfils and Uziel, 1987; Bonfils et al., 1988a]. This observation suggests a mechanical origin of TEOAE [Kemp, 1978]. The visual detection threshold is influenced by the frequency

Table 10. Latency of TEOAE in normal human ears

	Latency in wavelength	Latency in ms at 1 kHz
Kemp [1978]	8–25	15
Kemp [1980b]	10	10
Wit and Ritsma [1980, 1983a]	11–18	11
Rutten [1980b]	7–15	10
Wilson [1980c]	10–20	10
Johnsen and Elberling [1982b]	7–17	11
Schloth [1982]	10–16	12
Norton and Neely [1985, 1987]	10–20	16

content of TEOAE. Highly tuned emission frequencies, such as synchronized SOAE frequencies, imply longer durations of TEOAE and purer waveforms, presumably leading to lower detection thresholds. Additionally, less energy may be needed to phase lock SOAE than to evoke emissions not already present [Wit and Ritsma, 1983a]. Therefore, it is not surprising that ears showing narrow frequency components in their TEOAE have clearly lower thresholds than ears without such components [Probst et al., 1986]. However, psychoacoustic thresholds were comparable in both groups of ears. Thus, a direct indication of individual psychoacoustic thresholds cannot be obtained by the measurement of TEOAE threshold.

Additionally, age was shown to influence the detection thresholds of TEOAE by Bonfils et al. [1988a]. These investigators examined different age groups. The detection threshold had similar values of around 0 dB HL up to an age of 40 years when related to a normal hearing level, and around −5 dB SL up to an age of 30 years when related to the subjective click thresholds. After these ages, threshold increased linearly at a rate of about 8 dB HL per decade. Since a significant reduction of prominent emission frequencies was found only at ages above 50 years [Bonfils et al., 1988a], elements other than a broader tuning of responses may contribute to this increase in TEOAE thresholds. A similar age-dependent reduction in the bandwidth of the broadly tuned TEOAE frequency component was found by the same investigators and, additionally, a high correlation between these two age-dependent reductions. A possible explanation of this age-related threshold increase could be some mechanical changes beginning at about age 40, presumably located within the cochlea and/or the middle ear. Thus, TEOAE may offer a new possibility for studying presbycusis.

However, similar to latency measurements, it remains to be demonstrated that measurements of TEOAE detection threshold are useful for clinical purposes. For screening, the most imminent practical use of

TEOAE, threshold measurements are probably not necessary [Kemp et al., 1986; Bray and Kemp, 1987].

4.2.7. Amplitude and Input-Output Function. The amplitude of TEOAE depends on stimulus level, number and frequencies of dominant emission frequencies, frequency response of the middle ear, and of the recording system coupled to the ear canal. Additionally, ill understood individual factors may also be important. In order to estimate the output energy of TEOAE, the measurement of a simple peak to peak amplitude will be useful in only a few cases of TEOAE dominated by a single frequency. In most instances, however, TEOAE are multifrequency responses with several emission frequencies showing different latencies, amplitudes, durations, and thresholds. Therefore, methods integrating either sound pressure [Kemp, 1978; Zwicker, 1983a] or power spectra [Probst et al., 1986] within specific time windows were used to estimate TEOAE output. The placement of the time window influences these measurements because of the different latencies and durations of the frequency components. Early time windows may include stimulus ringing. Late windows may exclude short-lasting frequency components and are dominated by emission frequencies with long durations, such as synchronized SOAE.

In view of these methodological difficulties, it is not surprising that the input-output (I/O) functions reported in the literature differ considerably. The first I/O function was reported by Kemp [1978], who fitted his data points to the square root of the stimulus level. Close inspection of these data points, however, could indicate a nearly linear growth up to a stimulus level of about -25 dB SPL/Hz (corresponding to about 13 dB HL) and a strong saturation above this level. A constant gain of the TEOAE below stimulus levels of 10–20 dB HL along with pronounced saturation beginning above this level were later found by several investigators [Wit and Ritsma, 1979; Kemp and Chum, 1980b; Wilson, 1980a; Schloth, 1982; Zwicker, 1983a]. Many of these investigators [Wilson, 1980c; Wit et al., 1981; Zwicker, 1983a] stressed major differences between individual ears, and Zwicker [1983a] showed that I/O functions with the abovementioned characteristics were mainly found in ears without SOAE. Spontaneous emissions may interfere nonlinearly with TEOAE at lower stimulus levels.

Nonlinear growth of TEOAE at stimulus levels of more than about 20–30 dB SL is generally agreed upon. Such growth is one of the most distinct characteristics of TEOAE and often used to identify these emissions. The practical importance of it is paramount. The exact growth of TEOAE at lower stimulus levels, and its practical importance, is less clear and probably individually quite different.

4.2.8. Right-Left Ear Correlations. The two ears of a single subject tend to show similar TEOAE in relation to waveform, number of dominant emission frequencies, duration, or detection threshold [Probst et al., 1986; Bonfils et al., 1988a]. Significant correlations of these characteristics between the two ears of subjects were found. These findings support some structural factor common to both ears involved in the generation of TEOAE. Conceivable structural features could be genetically determined irregularities of hair cell patterns in the organ of Corti or symmetrically acquired hair cell losses.

4.2.9. External Influences. Generally, similar findings of external influences on TEOAE were reported as those already discussed in SOAE. In most reports, it must be assumed that the experiments were conducted in ears with robust TEOAE, infering the presence of highly tuned emission frequencies. Therefore, a similarity between the findings in SOAE and TEOAE would be expected. However, the coexistence or absence of SOAE when examining TEOAE was seldom reported. For example, suppression tuning curves with similar characteristics as those of SOAE were measured by Kemp [1979a], Wilson [1980a], Wit and Ritsma [1980], and Schloth [1982].

Masking, the interference of one auditory stimulus with another, can be studied in an objective way using TEOAE. Specifically, a distinction between a generation of masking before or at the level of neural elements can be made and the time structures of masking may be revealed. Using TEOAE, it was demonstrated that forward masking is a neural effect [Kemp and Chum, 1980b; Zwicker, 1983b; Scherer, 1984] and that, on the other hand, simultaneous masking [Kemp, 1988], backward masking [Kemp and Chum, 1980b; Scherer, 1984], or masking period patterns [Zwicker, 1981a, 1983b; Zwicker et al., 1987] had similar influences on TEOAE and psychoacoustic measures and that, therefore, they are most probably produced at preneural, cochlear levels.

The effect of acoustic overstimulation by loud noises on TEOAE was studied by Kemp [1981, 1982, 1988] and Zwicker [1983b]. Kemp [1981, 1982] showed that overstimulation led to depressions of TEOAE in a frequency selective manner, and mainly involved the late or highly tuned frequency components, including synchronized SOAE. Psychoacoustically well-known findings, such as TTS and half-octave shifts, correlated well with the TEOAE changes [Kemp, 1982; Zwicker, 1983b]. During the restoration of normal functions, regulatory changes of TEOAE with overshooting could be demonstrated by Kemp [1981, 1982, 1986, 1988]. He also pointed out [1988] that OAE provide a unique opportunity to study such regulatory mechanisms in the cochlea.

Finally, the effect of aspirin on TEOAE was demonstrated by several investigators [Johnsen and Elberling, 1982a; Long et al., 1986; Long and Tubis, 1988]. When cumulative doses of this drug were administered [Long et al., 1986; Long and Tubis, 1988], spontaneous emissions were reduced first, followed by narrowly tuned frequency components of TEOAE. That aspirin can also reduce broadband, short components of TEOAE, is shown in the example of figure 1 (page 7).

4.3. Findings in Patients

For future clinical use, it is particularly important to establish relationships between TEOAE and hearing disorders of clinical populations. Since TEOAE are nearly always found in normal hearing ears, they are being considered as a tool for objective hearing evaluation, particularly for screening and threshold determination.

4.3.1. Sensorineural Hearing Loss.

Kemp [1978] was the first who examined ears with sensorineural hearing loss. He found no TEOAE in ears with hearing losses of more than 30 dB. Rutten [1980a] examined six ears with high-frequency hearing loss above 2 kHz and found TEOAE in all. However, the hearing threshold at the dominant emission frequency was always 15 dB or better. Hinz and von Wedel [1984] studied patients after sudden hearing losses. In a total of five ears, they found TEOAE only after partial or complete recovery of cochlear function, thereby demonstrating the possibility of reappearance of TEOAE. Another example of such reappearance after improvement of hearing threshold is shown in figure 9.

It also demonstrates the fact that TEOAE can be present in ears having some preservation of hearing at specific frequencies along with marked sensorineural hearing loss at other frequencies [Rutten, 1980a; Kemp et al., 1986; Probst et al., 1987]. What, then, is the exact relationship between sensorineural hearing loss and TEOAE? It is generally agreed that no TEOAE can be detected in ears with hearing loss of 40 dB or more at 1 kHz, of about 35 dB or more for mean threshold values at 0.5, 1, 2, and 4 kHz [Kemp et al., 1986; Probst et al., 1987; Stevens, 1988; Bonfils et al., 1988b, d; Collet and Morgon, 1988; Lutman and Fleming, 1988]. Therefore, there seems to exist an upper value of hearing loss, above which no TEOAE can be detected. This value depends on several parameters, including the definition of the psychoacoustic threshold, the definition of absence or presence of TEOAE, and technical details of recording methods. Table 11 summarizes values of psychoacoustic thresholds from the literature at which ears with sensorineural hearing loss were divided into two groups. Ears with hearing loss above that value did not show TEOAE in more than 95% of the ears, but they were nearly always present in ears with hearing losses below that value.

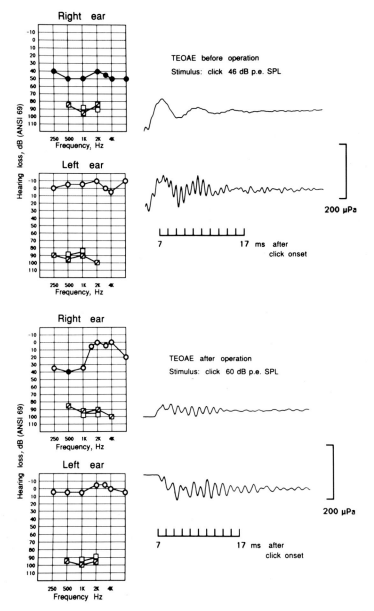

Fig. 9. Pure-tone audiograms, stapedial-reflex thresholds, and click-evoked emissions from a patient with Ménière's disease on the right side. Top: Audiograms and TEOAE recordings before surgery when a flat hearing loss of 40–50 dB was present in the right ear. No TEOAE is evident on this side, only low-frequency ringing of the stimulus. Bottom: Audiograms and TEOAE recordings nearly one year later, after the patient underwent an endolymphatic shunt operation. Reappearance of TEOAE can be recognized. Differences in the recordings on the left side are due to the use of different recording systems. Open dots: Air conduction, no masking. Filled dots: Masked air conduction. Squares: lpsilateral stapedial-reflex threshold. Crossed squares: Contralateral stapedial-reflex threshold.

Table 11. Upper values of psychoacoustic thresholds with TEOAE

	Number of ears examined	TEOAE 'threshold' dB nHL	Measured subjective threshold
Kemp [1978]	27	30	audiogram
Kemp et al. [1986]	88	15	1–2 kHz
Probst et al. [1987]	44	25	click
Bonfils et al. [1988a]	135	25	click
Stevens [1988]	38	18	click

The exact values in table 11 depended on the particular methods employed to measure behavoral thresholds. However, it can be safely stated that the presence of TEOAE indicate a hearing threshold of 30 dB HL or better, at least within a certain frequency range.

The determination of this frequency range is possible through the spectrum of the TEOAE [Kemp et al., 1986; Probst et al., 1987]. The frequency region between 1 and 2 kHz seems to be most important for the preservation of TEOAE [Kemp et al., 1986; Probst et al., 1987; Collet and Morgon, 1988]. However, with click-evoked emissions no information is obtained about other frequency ranges than those contained in the TEOAE spectrum, and no prediction about the hearing threshold outside this spectrum is possible [Probst et al., 1987; Lutman and Fleming, 1988]. The TEOAE spectrum shows wide variations even in the normal ear [Probst et al., 1986], and it does not allow conclusions concerning the pattern of hearing loss. The use of more frequency-specific tonebursts as stimuli may be helpful [Probst et al., 1986; Norton and Neely, 1987], but results with these stimuli from patients are still lacking.

Another important variable in the generation of TEOAE, apart from hearing thresholds, may be the etiology of the hearing disorder. Click-evoked emissions were reported to be present in ears with Ménière's disease, despite a hearing threshold above 40 dB HL [Bonfils et al., 1988d]. Kemp et al. [1986] reported similar findings, but a change in hearing thresholds could not be excluded, since the audiogram and TEOAE testing were done at different dates. The fact that TEOAE can reappear in ears with improved hearing thresholds was already demonstrated in figure 9. Additionally, amplitude changes of TEOAE in ears with Ménière's disease after glycerol administration were reported by Bonfils et al. [1988d], Uziel and Bonfils [1988], and Collet and Morgon [1988]. However, as a group, ears with Ménière's disease did not show significantly different TEOAE characteristics as compared to ears with other forms of sensorineural hearing loss [Kemp et al., 1986; Probst et al., 1987; Uziel and Bonfils, 1988].

Noise-induced high-frequency hearing loss may lead to a reduction of TEOAE incidence and of the number of dominant emission frequencies per ear [Probst et al., 1987]. When a group of ears with presumably noise-induced hearing loss was compared to a group of ears with similar hearing losses not related to noise, significantly fewer TEOAE were found in the noise-induced damage group. This finding could indicate that TEOAE testing may detect the presence of widespread, subclinical loss of outer hair cells, which was demonstrated in ears with noise-induced hearing loss [Bohne and Clark, 1982; Hawkins and Johnsen, 1976].

Ears with retrocochlear hearing loss due to acoustic neuromas were studied by Kemp et al. [1986] and Bonfils et al. [1988e]. Some 30 patients were tested and TEOAE were detected in only about a third of the involved ears. Thus, the hearing loss in acoustic neuromas must be associated in a high percentage with cochlear damages, induced through either vascular or efferent influences. Therefore, the hope of diagnosing retrocochlear hearing loss through the demonstration of preserved TEOAE, along with significant hearing threshold loss, was not realized.

In conclusion, TEOAE are not dependent on an entirely intact cochlear function, but relative preservation in some frequency regions suffices. The frequency range with the most important, but not exclusive, influence is between 1 and 2 kHz. The critical hearing loss for TEOAE preservation is about 25–30 dB HL. Moreover, loss of TEOAE may be reversible. These findings may be modified by different etiologies of sensorineural hearing loss. Ménière's disease may show relative preservation of TEOAE, while noise-induced hearing loss may show a relative loss.

4.3.2. Infants. One possible conclusion from the results in normal and pathological ears is that the testing of TEOAE 'does not quantify hearing loss, it detects its presence' [Kemp et al., 1986]. Therefore, TEOAE may be an ideal means for screening purposes, and infants would be a primary group in which such objective screening is desirable. Indeed, technical developments of TEOAE testing has been directed to overcome the special problems associated with infants and small children [Kemp et al., 1986; Bray and Kemp, 1987]. One hundred normal neonates were examined by Johnsen et al. [1983, 1988]. In all but one ear, TEOAE to a 2-kHz half-sinusoidal click were found. Therefore, the incidence of TEOAE was essentially the same as in adults. These results were later confirmed by Bray and Kemp [1987], Stevens et al. [1987], and Bonfils et al. [1988c]. The characteristics of TEOAE in neonates appear to be similar to those in adults, with the possible exception of the frequency spectrum, which may show higher averages [Johnsen et al., 1988; Bray and Kemp, 1987; Bonfils et al., 1988c].

Testing for TEOAE in various risk groups and in children with hearing losses was reported by Bray and Kemp [1987], Stevens et al. [1987, 1988], Bonfils et al. [1988c], Lutman and Fleming [1988], and Thornton [1988]. A good correlation between the findings of testing for auditory brainstem responses (ABR) and TEOAE testing was noted in infants requiring special neonatal care [Stevens et al., 1987, 1988; Bonfils et al., 1988c]. Sensitivity of TEOAE as a screening device in this special group was noted to be almost 100% by all of the above-mentioned investigators. The specificity, however, is not yet clear, since its assessment is only possible by long-term follow-up studies. Such studies are under way [Stevens et al., 1988; Lutman and Fleming, 1988; Thornton, 1988]. Stevens et al. [1988] reported on 346 babies. Eighty percent of them passed a first TEOAE test (normal newborns 96%). Combined with ABR testing, only 8% failed. Twelve babies were considered on retesting to be at a high risk of hearing impairment, which would indicate a specificity of 83% for TEOAE testing alone, or 91% when combined with ABR. However, follow-up was not complete and these figures have to be considered preliminary. A similar specificity of 73%, with the same reservations, was reported by Lutman and Fleming [1988].

A logical strategy for infant screening would be to first test TEOAE. With automated, special noise-rejecting equipment [Bray and Kemp, 1987], this test could be carried out in a few minutes. Based on the available results in adults and children, the demonstration of TEOAE can safely be expected to indicate relative normal hearing at certain frequency ranges. Some forms of mild or moderate hearing loss may be missed and no discrete frequency specific information can be obtained. However, children needing special measures immediately, like hearing aids and/or special education, should be recognized. If the infant fails the screening test for TEOAE, more time consuming methods like ABR testing, possibly combined with impedance audiometry, or behavioral measurements should follow.

4.4. Findings in Animals

Similar to the findings in SOAE, TEOAE were found irregularly and, in most species, with considerably lower incidences than in human ears. Table 12 summarizes the reports found in the literature.

Only bats (*Pteronotus parnelli*) showed TEOAE in every instance [Kössl and Vater, 1985]. The frequencies of these TEOAE were located in the ultrasound spectrum around 62 kHz. Otherwise, their general properties were remarkably similar to those of human TEOAE. The regular demonstration of TEOAE makes it highly unlikely that a pathological substratum is responsible for the generation of these emissions in bats. Indeed, a

Table 12. Incidence of TEOAE reported in different species

	Species	TEOAE	Number of tested ears	Number of ears with TEOAE	%
Anderson [1980]	primate	+	18 (?)	11	61
Yates and Bishop [1979]	guinea pig	−	?	0	0
Wit and Ritsma [1980]	guinea pig	−	?	0	0
Wilson [1980c]; Wilson and Evans [1983]	cat	+	10	3	30
Schmiedt and Adams [1981]	gerbil	−	28	0	0
	guinea pig	−	4	0	0
Zwicker and Manley [1981]	guinea pig	+	12	5	42
Wit and Kahman [1982]	primate	+	10	7	70
Palmer and Wilson [1982]	frog	+	?	?	
Kössl and Vater [1985]	bat	+	15	15	100
Strack [1986]	caiman	−	7	0	0
Manley et al. [1987]	starling	−	6	0	0

correlation of TEOAE to the high frequency orientation call and to morphological specializations of the bat cochlea could be demonstrated.

Primates showed TEOAE with a relatively high incidence of 65% [Anderson, 1980; Wit and Kahmann, 1982]. These results were obtained in different species (*M. irus, Erythrocebus patas, M. nemestrina, M. mulatta*). Again, the general properties of the TEOAE were similar to those found in human, including the presence of dominant emission frequencies between 1 and 4.5 kHz and the same general form of the I/O functions. However, amplitudes were somewhat smaller and latencies somewhat shorter. Detailed measures of TEOAE in a rhesus monkey with SOAE were reported by Martin et al. [1988]. An example of the TEOAE to a click stimulus in this monkey along with an emission from a human ear are depicted in figure 10. The remarkable similarity of these two TEOAE is evident. Both emissions have a long duration, are dominated by a single frequency, and show amplitude modulations at the beginning as a sign of additional emission frequencies.

In rodents, TEOAE are found only as the exception and not as a rule. Zwicker and Manley [1981] were the only investigators demonstrating TEOAE in guinea pigs. Other investigators [Yates and Bishop, 1979; Wit and Ritsma, 1980; Schmiedt and Adams, 1981] could not replicate this finding, even when similar methods to those used by Zwicker and Manley [1981] were employed [Schmiedt and Adams, 1981]. An explanation for these discrepancies is not evident.

In conclusion, while TEOAE seem to be a general property in ears of humans and, possibly, of bats, they are much less common in other

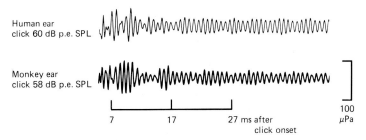

Fig. 10. Comparison of TEOAE to a click stimulus recorded in a human ear (top) and a monkey ear (bottom). Similarities include long durations, dominant emission-frequencies, and amplitude modulations.

mammals, with old world monkeys showing them most regularly in about 60% of ears. They are generally missing in rodents. If present, TEOAE in animals are, however, remarkably similar to those found in human ears.

5. Stimulus-Frequency Otoacoustic Emissions

SFOAE are generated during a continuous stimulation with a single pure-tone, and they represent a steady-state, in contrast to TEOAE. The SFOAE consist of additional acoustic energy at the stimulus frequency. The relative amplitude in proportion to the stimulus generally grows nonlinearly with decreasing stimulus intensities. Kemp and Chum [1980a] were the first to describe this class of OAE.

5.1. Methods of Recording

Similar acoustic probes are used for the recording of SFOAE as those described for the TEOAE. The stimulus consists of a pure tone which is, in most instances, swept over a certain frequency range. The stimulus level within the ear canal is measured with a narrowband filtering device. Stimulus-frequency emissions can be demonstrated through manipulations of either stimulus frequency and/or stimulus level. Alternatively, one can also use the addition of a suppressing tone. Analog filters, heterodyne filters, of FFT may be used for measuring the stimulus level.

Sweeping of the stimulus frequency leads to phase changes between the evoked emissions and the stimulus. This, in turn leads to frequency regions with enhanced sound pressure level and adjacent regions with depressed levels which can be recorded as peaks and valleys when the measuring frequency of the filter is swept synchronously to the stimulus. Additionally, the use of different stimulus levels allows differentiation between SFOAE and variations of the sound pressure level caused by ear canal resonances.

The emissions show saturation and are relatively small when louder stimulus levels are used and relatively large at levels near the threshold. The subtraction of scaled values obtained with high and low level stimuli cancels the resonant changes of the sound pressure levels, leaving the emission component [Kemp and Chum, 1980a; Schloth, 1982]. This component can alternatively be measured by the addition of a suppressing tone with a frequency close to the stimulus [Kemp and Brown, 1983a].

The introduction of an artifact rejection system is not as straightforward as in recording systems for TEOAE. Such a system is conceivable with special data processing like digital averaging of discrete measuring points along a frequency axis. However, to my knowledge, no such systems have, to date, been used clinically.

5.2. Findings in Normal Human Subjects

Many characteristics of SFOAE of human ears are very similar to those of TEOAE, though the former are produced by a steady stimulus and not by transient stimulation. The main similarities concern the strong saturation of the emissions with moderately intense stimuli, the incidence, and the main frequency ranges where they occur. These similarities point to a generation of SFOAE and TEOAE that possibly shares common mechanisms.

5.2.1. Incidence.
The incidence of SFOAE was not systematically studied in human ears. Kemp and Chum [1980a] examined eight ears of six subjects and found SFOAE in seven. Rutten and Buisman [1983] reported SFOAE in 17 ears of ten subjects. Zwicker and Schloth [1984] found SFOAE in seven of ten subjects, in six of them at multiple frequencies. Dallmayr [1987] reported SFOAE in 18 of 20 ears. Overall, 49 of 55 ears, or 89%, showed SFOAE.

This figure is somewhat lower than the incidence of TEOAE. It seems that SFOAE may be difficult to record in ears with very short TEOAE showing only broadly tuned frequencies. Further evidence for this statement will be discussed later.

5.2.2. Frequency.
If a stimulus with sweeping frequency is used, typical nonlinear peaks and valleys indicate the presence of SFOAE. The frequencies of these peaks, or valleys, are constant for an individual ear. However, each ear shows an individual pattern of the numbers and frequencies of these peaks. Figure 11 represents an example of SFOAE in a human ear. At least five peaks, indicating five emission frequencies, can be recognized.

There is evidence [Kemp and Chum, 1980a; Rutten and Buisman, 1983; Zwicker and Schloth, 1984] that these peaks and valleys are generated

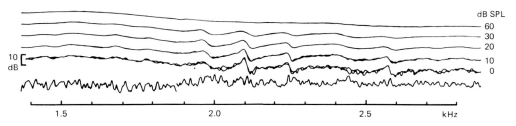

Fig. 11. Sound pressure level in a human ear canal measured during a stimulation with several intensities and sweeping frequency in the range 1.4–2.8 kHz. The top curve, recorded with 60 dB SPL, represents the frequency response of the acoustic system (SFOAE are saturated). Beginning with 30 dB SPL, perturbations of the baseline can be noted, indicating emission frequencies. Bottom curve: No stimulus condition.

by fixed emission frequencies corresponding to fixed places on the basilar membrane. Through phase changes, the interaction of the fixed emission frequency and the changing stimulus frequency leads to the generation of the typical perturbations of the measured sound level.

The same emission frequencies could be found in SFOAE as in TEOAE or in SOAE [Rutten and Buisman, 1983]. The number of emission frequencies and their frequency ranges were highly similar to those found in TEOAE [Rutten and Buisman, 1983]. That SFOAE can be generated by spontaneously oscillating emission frequencies was demonstrated by bi-modal amplitude histograms of SFOAE [Divenyi, 1986]. Moreover, the average distance between two adjacent emission frequencies were also similar to those found for TEOAE or SOAE [Zwicker and Schloth, 1984; Dallmayr, 1987]. Zwicker and Schloth [1984] examined the interpeak distance in seven normal hearing subjects. An increase of the average distance from 50 Hz at 0.5 kHz to 150 Hz at 2.5 kHz was found. However, the individual variability was quite large. Dallmayr [1987] reported the most frequent distance to be around 0.08 octaves, which corresponds to 80 Hz at 1 kHz. Zwicker and Schloth [1984] pointed out that these distances resemble the critical bandwidth of psychoacoustical measurements. A theoretical connection between these two phenomena is, however, lacking.

It is unclear if a second emission component of SFOAE, not linked to fixed frequencies, can be found in human ears. If present, this would mean that SFOAE could be recorded at all frequencies over a certain frequency range, regardless whether fixed emission frequencies are located within this range or not. Kemp and Chum [1980a] and Dallmayr [1987] presented some evidence for such a component without definitely demonstrating it. Other investigations [Kemp and Brown, 1983a, b; Zwicker and Schloth, 1984; Kemp, 1986] could not find such a component. It must be concluded that an SFOAE component not linked to fixed emission frequencies must be very small and difficult to detect in human ears, if it is present at all.

5.2.3. Latency. The latency of SFOAE can be determined with phase measurements as group latency. Several investigators reported similar latencies of around ten wavelenghts [Kemp and Chum, 1980a; Schloth, 1982; Kemp and Brown, 1983a]. Absolute latencies were measured with special averaging techniques by Dallmayr [1987]. He found a latency for appearance of SFOAE of about 7 ms and, thereafter, an exponential growth with a time constant of about 5 ms. Therefore, the latencies of SFOAE are also similar to those of TEOAE. These latencies, however, were only measured for SFOAE generated by fixed emission frequencies. There is no information about latencies of a possible second SFOAE component in human ear.

5.2.4. Amplitude and Input-Output Function. The sound pressure levels of SFOAE vary between -20 and $+10$ dB SPL [Kemp and Chum, 1980a; Schloth, 1982; Rutten and Buisman, 1983; Dallmayr, 1987]. As already mentioned, there is a strong saturation at moderate stimulus levels, but different shapes of the entire I/O functions were reported. Rutten and Buisman [1983] distinguished different functions for emission frequencies corresponding to SOAE compared to those where no SOAE were present. Highly irregular functions were found in connection with SOAE. Other emission frequencies showed a gain of around two thirds at lower stimulus levels, and an additional compressive component was found at higher stimulus levels in about half of these SFOAE. A similar gain of 0.6 was reported by Kemp and Brown [1983a] in the stimulus range of 10–70 dB SPL. Zwicker and Schloth [1984], however, reported I/O functions similar to those in TEOAE, i.e. a gain of nearly one up to stimulus levels of about 20 dB SL, followed by a strong compression at higher levels. Dallmayr [1987] measured essentially the same I/O functions as Zwicker and Schloth [1984].

5.2.5. Comparison to Transiently Evoked Emissions. Stimulus-frequency emissions of human ears were studied in considerably less detail than TEOAE. Moreover, no reports about the behavior of SFOAE in pathological ears are available. All findings indicate, however, that many properties of SFOAE resemble those of TEOAE and a common cochlear origin is conceivable. The findings of acoustic suppressions of SFOAE reported by Kemp and Chum [1980a] and by Dallmayr [1987] can be regarded as further evidence for the similarity of SFOAE and TEOAE, since they resembled those of TEOAE in general and detailed properties.

Whereas in TEOAE, a broadband click evokes several different emission frequencies simultaneously and in a transient way, the same emission frequencies seem to be evoked separately and successively in SFOAE. Since TEOAE show linear superpositions in time [Zwicker, 1983a] and frequency domain [Elberling et al., 1985; Probst et al., 1986], no substantial differences between these two stimulus forms should be expected. Indeed, the many similarities already discussed support this assumption. Additionally, direct comparisons of the two emission forms [Zwicker and Schloth, 1984; Long and Tubis, 1988] in the same ear further confirm the assumption.

5.3. Findings in Animals

Stimulus-frequency emissions could be demonstrated in several species with different cochlear systems dissimilar in major functional aspects. Table 13 summarizes the species, the measured SFOAE levels, and special attributes concerning the examinations or the species.

5.3.1. Differences to Human Stimulus-Frequency Emissions. Many of the SFOAE listed in table 13 differ substantially from human SFOAE in important characteristics. These differences mainly concern findings of the frequency range, latency, and amplitude.

Two components of SFOAE could be distinguished in the gerbil [Kemp and Brown, 1983a; Kemp, 1986]. The first component showed certain similarities to the SFOAE of human ears. However, it was not regularly found, its amplitude was small, the latency was only 2–5 wavelengths, and it grew with a gain of only 0.3. A second SFOAE component was detected at stimulus levels above 40 dB SPL which occurred with a latency of only 0.3 wavelength and which grew with a gain of 1.7 without showing saturation. These characteristics were never found in human SFOAE, but they resemble those of SFOAE in the alligator lizard [Rosowski et al., 1984a]. These animals showed a similar nonlinear component with stimulations above 70 dB SPL. Additionally, the guinea pig exhibited a similar component [Kemp and Souter, 1988] which could be influenced by weak stimulations of the efferent system innervating the cochlea.

Less dissimilarities to human SFOAE than in rodents or alligator lizards were found in the SFOAE of caimans [Strack, 1986] and starlings [Manley et al., 1987]. The SFOAE of these two species resembled each other quite closely. Manley et al. [1987] found emissions in 34 (61%) of 56 starling ears, Strack [1986] in four of five caiman ears. The amplitudes were between −40 and +2 dB SPL for starlings, and between −35 and +5 dB SPL for caimans. An average of three peaks and valleys in the frequency range of 1–5.5 kHz were found in starlings, compared to an

Table 13. SFOAE reported in animals

	Species	Amplitude in dB SPL	Remarks
Palmer and Wilson [1982]	frog	<20	no basilar membrane
Kemp and Brown [1983a]	gerbil	−5/10−40	two components
Rosowski et al. [1984a]	alligator lizard	40	no traveling wave
Kössl and Vater [1985]	bat	60	frequency at 62 kHz
Strack [1986]	caiman	5	no TEOAE
Manley et al. [1987]	starling	<2	no TEOAE
Martin et al. [1988]	primate	<20	SOAE present

average of four peaks in the range of 0.4–2.2 kHz in caimans. Suppression tuning curves of both species were comparable to those obtained in humans. Thus, the main difference to human SFOAE concerns the smaller amplitudes. Additionally, the bandwidth of SFOAE was 200 Hz in both species and, therefore, broader than those in humans, where the bandwidth was typically around 40 Hz [Zwicker and Schloth, 1984]. Similar bandwidths of 200 Hz were found in frogs [Palmer and Wilson, 1982], but these animals showed SFOAE of up to 20 dB SPL.

In conclusion, SFOAE of several species can differ considerably from each other and from those found in human ears. In view of these differences and of the anatomically different cochleas of these species, it is probable that more than one functional process leads to the generation of these emissions. However, nonlinearities seem to be a functional component of many cochlear systems.

5.3.2. Similarities to Human Stimulus-Frequency Emissions. Human SFOAE are dominated by fixed emission frequencies. The same can be stated for SFOAE of bats [Kössl and Vater, 1985] and primates [Martin et al., 1988]. In all ears of 15 bats, SFOAE at about 62 or 0.7 kHz above the orientation cry were found [Kössl and Vater, 1985], which was also the frequency of TEOAE. Apart from the higher frequency and from a larger amplitude of about 65 dB SPL, the characteristics of these SFOAE, especially their I/O functions, resembled those found in human SFOAE.

Even more similarities to human SFOAE were found in a detailed study of these emissions from a nonhuman primate with SOAE [Martin et al., 1988]. Stable, multiple peaks were found that corresponded to emission frequencies of either SOAE or TEOAE. An example of SFOAE of this monkey is shown in figure 12.

The similarities to human SFOAE not only included the general form, but also the frequency range, the frequency distances between the peaks,

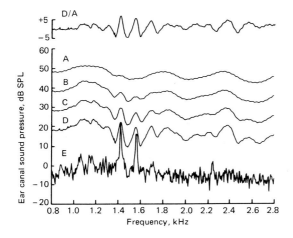

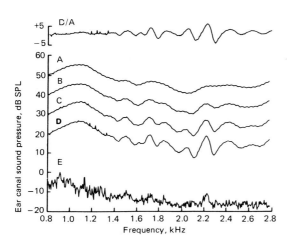

Fig. 12. Stimulus-frequency emissions and registration of SOAE following immediately (bottom curve, no stimulation). *a* Right ear, *b* left ear. Top curve D/A: Difference between curve A, corresponding to the loudest stimulation with saturation of SFOAE, and curve D, corresponding to the weakest stimulation with clear SFOAE. The linear elements are cancelled in the difference curve D/A. From Martin et al. [1988], with permission of the publisher.

the amplitudes, and their response to aspirin. Fixed emission frequencies with much the same characteristics as those found in human ears dominated the OAE of this monkey. Therefore, its cochlea may serve as a model of the majority of normal human ears, which also show SFOAE, TEOAE, and sometimes SOAE dominated by fixed emission frequencies. Indeed, as will be discussed later, the histological examination of these monkey ears

[Lonsbury-Martin et al., 1988b] provided many insights with possible implications concerning the OAE generation in human ears.

6. Otoacoustic Emissions of Distortion Products

DP are phenomena of many physical systems. They are generated by nonlinear elements, which distort the signal and thereby create additional frequencies. The presence of DP in the human auditory system has been known for many years [Helmholtz, 1870; Békésy, 1934]. Helmholtz [1870] thought that these distortions were generated in the most obvious mechanical system known to him, namely the middle ear. Investigations by Békésy [1934] and Wever et al. [1940] seemed to confirm that DP of the auditory system were generated by overdriving the mechanical system at high levels. Later, mainly psychoacoustical measurements [Zwicker, 1955; Plomp, 1965; Goldstein, 1967; Wenner, 1968] proved the existence of DP, and thus of nonlinear elements, in the auditory system at medium level stimuli. Goldstein [1967] proposed the basilar membrane as the locus of generation.

Shortly after the discovery of TEOAE [Kemp, 1978], OAE linked to DP were demonstrated in human ears [Kemp, 1979a]. They consisted of acoustic energy at specific frequencies which were not detectable in the spectrum of the acoustic stimulus above the noise floor. The stimulus frequencies are called the primaries ($f_1 < f_2 < f_3$ etc.), and the frequencies of DP are related to them by mathematical formulas. In human ears, as well as in the ears of many animal species, the difference intermodulation DP at the frequency of $2f_1 - f_2$ is the most prominent OAE, and it is also the most thoroughly examined. The amplitude of DPOAE is dependent on the amplitudes of the primary stimuli. While many rodents exhibit DPOAE of approximatley 40 dB smaller than the stimulus levels, this value amounts to 60 dB or more in human ears.

6.1. Methods of Recording

A primary concern when measuring DPOAE, especially in human ears, is the distinction between biologically produced DP and those related to the equipment used for stimulation and measuring OAE. Therefore, a system with linear characteristics in the measuring range is required. The dynamic range of such a system should reach about 80 dB in the audiofrequency range. Only high quality systems will meet these requirements, and special care must be taken because each system may produce unforeseen nonlinearities in acoustic probes coupled to the ear canal in a closed fashion.

Since two pure tones are the most widely used stimuli for measuring DPOAE, a mixture of the sine waves is necessary. This can be accomplished either electronically using only one transducer, or acoustically after generating the tones with two transducers. Generally, the second method is less prone to nonlinear interactions. The acoustic probe may have only one speaker port for either an electronically mixed signal or an acoustically mixed signal delivered by a Y-tube. Alternatively, it can contain two separate stimulus ports providing mixture of the stimulus within the ear canal. The measurement of the DPOAE at a preselected frequency can be done by narrowband filtering devices, such as digital filters using FFT, heterodyne filters, or analog filters.

6.2. Findings in Normal Human Subjects

Otoacoustic emissions of DP are methodologically difficult to measure in human ears because of their relatively small amplitudes. This may be one of the reasons that DPOAE have not been examined in human ears as extensively as other classes of OAE. An additional difficulty is represented by the multitude of parameters that have to be considered and that can be varied, e.g. the frequency ratio of the primaries, their level ratio, the particular DP frequency to be measured, and the frequency ranges where the primaries, the DP, and the DP generation site are located. Emissions of DP in human ears were almost exclusively measured at the frequency of $2f_1-f_2$. From a number of studies [Zwicker, 1955, 1979b, 1980a, b, 1981b; Goldstein, 1967; Smoorenburg, 1972; Hall, 1972; Weber and Mellert, 1975; Zurek and Leshowitz, 1976; Humes, 1983, 1985], the following psychoacoustical properties of this particular DP were known: (1) The amplitude of the DP at $2f_1-f_2$ showed a variability of 10–20 dB. The amplitude was found to be dependent on the relations of the frequencies and levels of the two primaries. Small frequency ratios of f_2/f_1 gave generally larger DP amplitudes than widely spaced primaries. Additionally, the largest amplitudes were obtained when the level of the lower-frequency primary (f_1) was 5–10 dB higher than the higher-frequency primary (f_2). (2) When equal level primaries were used, the I/O function of the DP amplitude generally grew linearly with a slope of approximately 1, up to a stimulus level of 60–70 dB SPL. Saturation was found in most cases with higher stimulus levels. (3) Nonmonotonous individual I/O functions were sometimes found, especially with f_2/f_1 ratios of more than 1.25. (4) The DP was found psychoacoustically in most normal hearing subjects in the frequency range of 0.5–5 kHz with a maximum incidence between 1 and 2 kHz.

Several of these findings were confirmed for DPOAE at $2f_1-f_2$ as well. However, some differences were reported [Wilson, 1980d; Furst et al., 1988]. Most of these can be explained by confounding influences of SOAE and by the fact that psychoacoustical perception takes place at regions of the basilar membrane apical to the stimulus frequencies, whereas DPOAE are dependent on a basal transmission of the signal. The amplitudes of DPOAE measured in the ear canal have to be regarded as a summation product of many vibrations at the base of the basilar membrane near the stapes, similar to CM measured at the round window [Zwicker, 1980a; Kemp and Brown, 1984; Matthews and Molnar, 1986].

6.2.1. Incidence. There is growing evidence that DPOAE are a general property of normal human ears, though this is not generally acknowledged in the literature [Furst and Lapid, 1988]. Kemp et al. [1986] reported DPOAE in all of 14 normal ears, Lonsbury-Martin et al. [1988a] in 44 ears, and Harris and Glattke [1988] in 20 subjects. These findings and our own experience with 113 normal ears [Probst et al., 1989] indicate that DPOAE can be recorded in well over 90% of normal ears. The frequency range where these emissions could be reliably detected was between 1 and 6 kHz with respect to the geometric mean of f_1 and f_2. Therefore, DPOAE seem to be present in the same frequency range as other classes of OAE. Again, a possible explanation could be the frequency range of the most effective reverse middle ear transmission.

6.2.2. Amplitude. The amplitude of DPOAE is dependent on several factors, including the level and frequency of the primaries, their ratios, and the individual ear. If the DPOAE frequency coincides with a SOAE or a dominant emission frequency of TEOAE, the amplitude of the DPOAE can be relatively large [Wilson, 1980d; Wit et al., 1981; Schloth, 1982; Furst et al., 1988; Wier et al., 1988]. Through enhancement by place-fixed emission frequencies, the amplitude can reach levels of only 10–20 dB smaller than the primaries. This effect is limited to a narrow frequency range [Wit et al., 1981], and it is most pronounced with f_2/f_1 ratios of less than 1.25. Apart from these special circumstances, the DPOAE amplitude in human ears is approximatley 60 dB smaller than the primaries [Schloth, 1982; Kemp and Brown, 1983a, b; Brown and Kemp, 1984; Kemp et al., 1986; Harris et al., 1987; Harris and Glattke, 1988; Lonsbury-Martin et al., 1988a].

The frequency distance between the two primaries is crucially important. Wilson [1980d] found the largest amplitudes with f_2/f_1 ratios between 1.1 and 1.2. However, these measurements were done at a strong emission frequency and, since Kemp [1986] showed that such low-frequency ratios tend to enhance individual place-fixed emission patterns, they may not be representative. Kemp and Brown [1983a] reported maximal amplitudes in six ears at f_2/f_1 ratios of 1.25. A similar ratio of 1.22 was reported by Harris et al. [1987] as most effective. The values of several stimulus conditions were averaged. These investigators also described systematic relationships of f_2/f_1 ratios to DP frequencies and to stimulus levels. Maximal amplitudes were obtained with higher ratios at low DP frequencies and at relatively high stimulus levels as opposed to high DP frequencies or low stimulus levels.

The level ratio of f_1 and f_2 has been less thoroughly examined in human ears. However, findings in animals and theoretical considerations point to levels $f_1 > f_2$ as most effective with differences of 5–10 dB. Schloth [1982] confirmed this level ratio in a single ear.

6.2.3. Threshold and Input-Output Function. Thresholds of DPOAE depend almost entirely on the noise floor and the sensitivity of the measuring equipment. Lonsbury-Martin et al. [1988a] reported 'thresholds' of 3 dB above the noise floor at 35–45 dB SPL. Much lower thresholds, down to 5 dB SPL, were found when measurements were taken near or at strong emission frequencies [Wilson, 1980d; Schloth, 1982; Burns et al., 1984b; Wier et al., 1988].

Wilson [1980d] and Schloth [1982] each measured I/O functions for three ears. Both investigators examined DPOAE at strong emission frequencies and made comparisons to psychoacoustical measurements. While Wilson [1980d] obtained widely differing functions for several f_2/f_1 ratios, Schloth [1982] found a slope of 1 when both primaries were at the same level. No clear differences between psychoacoustical and otoacoustical findings were found by either investigator.

Averaged I/O functions of 44 normal ears were reported by Lonsbury-Martin et al. [1988a]. With respect to the geometric mean frequencies of the primaries, the functions were generally less steep at lower frequencies of 1–3 kHz than at higher frequencies of 3–8 kHz, and they generally did not reach slopes of 1.

6.2.4. Latency. The latency of DPOAE can be defined by phase measurements. A systematic relation between phase and f_2/f_1 ratios was found by Wilson [1980d] and Kemp and Brown [Kemp and Brown, 1983a, b; Kemp, 1986]. The latency was much shorter with high rather than with low ratios. Wilson reported a latency of about half a cycle for ratios of 1.3, and of two and a half cycles for ratios of 1.1. Kemp [1986] summarized the phase measurements made in his laboratory. The phase was found to be nearly constant with slow frequency sweeps of the primaries at a fixed f_2/f_1 ratio of about 1.3, indicating a very short group latency. Group latencies increased with decreasing f_2/f_1 ratios and latencies up to 8 ms were measured. In addition, latency appeared to decrease slightly with increasing stimulus levels.

These findings indicate, as was pointed out by Kemp [1986], that two different generation mechanisms may be at work for DPOAE, a mechanism with similar latencies as those found in TEOAE for low level stimuli with primaries of frequencies close together, and a short latency mechanism with higher stimuli and larger f_2/f_1 ratios.

6.2.5. External Influences. Two different external influences on DPOAE were tested in human ears, acoustic suppression and aspirin. Suppression measurements were reported by Brown and Kemp [Brown and Kemp, 1983, 1984; Kemp and Brown, 1983a]. The general forms of the suppression tuning curves were similar to those found with other OAE classes. For $2f_1-f_2$, the maximum of suppression was always in the frequency range between the primaries and not around the DP frequency, indicating the generation of these DPOAE at a frequency place between the primaries. However, complex tuning curves with several minima were measured in most instances. Additionally, Brown and Kemp [1983, 1984] noted quite similar suppression tuning curves between human and gerbil ears.

The influence of aspirin was examined by Wier et al. [1988]. Aspirin ingestion clearly induced less amplitude reduction of DPOAE than the amount observed in SOAE in the same ears. Additionally, the reductions were less pronounced or even absent at higher primary levels. However, the enhancing influence of the SOAE frequency place on DPOAE amplitude was nearly unchanged by aspirin, even if SOAE were no longer detectable. Therefore, while the dissociation of the response to aspirin between SOAE and DPOAE indicated different generation mechanisms for these emissions, the constant influence of the SOAE frequency place suggested a close interrelation of the two emission types, at least at the DP frequency place.

6.2.6. Relation to Other Otoacoustic Emissions. Fixed emission frequencies of an individual ear, found either as SOAE, TEOAE, or SFOAE, can have an influence on the DPOAE amplitudes [Kemp, 1979a; Wilson, 1980d; Wit et al., 1981; Schloth, 1982; Kemp and Brown, 1983b; Burns et al., 1984b; Kemp, 1986; Wier et al., 1988; Furst et al., 1988]. Generally, a strong enhancing effect on the DPOAE amplitude could be found at fixed emission frequencies. This influence was shown to decrease with increasing stimulus levels [Kemp and Brown, 1983a; Kemp, 1986; Wier et al., 1988] and with increasing f_2/f_1 ratios [Wilson, 1980d; Kemp, 1986; Furst et al., 1988].

Several investigators [Burns et al., 1984b; Jones et al., 1986; Frick and Matthies, 1988] reported the existence of DPOAE evoked by two coexisting SOAE, representing examples of particularly low stimulus levels. However, the presence of an additional fixed emission frequency at the DPOAE place seemed to be necessary for the generation of these DPOAE. They are relatively rare, even in ears with multiple SOAE. Burns et al. [1984b] and

Jones et al. [1986] found 11 such DPOAE at $2f_1-f_2$ in eight ears of seven subjects. The amplitudes of these 'DP-SOAE' were 10–15 dB smaller than those of the SOAE that acted as the lower-frequency primary, but it could be equal in amplitude or even bigger than the higher-frequency primary SOAE. This finding confirms the psychoacoustical result that the largest DP amplitudes are generally obtained with levels $f_1 > f_2$. Frick and Matthies [1988] reported one ear with a possible DP-SOAE at f_2-f_1.

The strong influence of fixed emission frequencies on DPOAE amplitudes may be considered unexpected since the generation site of the DPOAE $2f_1-f_2$ is generally believed to be near the primaries [Kim et al., 1980; Siegel et al., 1982; Brown and Kemp, 1984; Dolan and Abbas, 1985a; Matthews and Molnar, 1986; Zwicker, 1986c; Lonsbury-Martin et al., 1987]. However, the DP itself probably acts as a weak stimulus and may induce, as a single frequency stimulus, stimulus-frequency-like emissions at the DP site. The fact that DP can be clearly audible could support this assumption. Since the amplifying effect of the OAE mechanism at fixed frequencies is thought to be strongest near the threshold, even a very low stimulus level, such as a 'DP stimulus', can be expected to evoke emissions.

6.3. Findings in Patients

Few results of DPOAE in pathological ears have been published. Kemp et al. [1986] reported three examples of DPOAE measurements in ears with high-frequency hearing loss. The DPOAE amplitudes were significantly smaller than normal values at frequencies where hearing thresholds were higher than 30 dB. However, DPOAE were still present in most instances and the frequency relations were not always straightforward.

Additional examples were reported by Franklin et al. [1988], who could objectively detect a 20-dB noise-induced impairment and a 10-dB hearing improvement in a case of suspected Ménière's disease following a glycerol test.

Systematic results in 20 patients with high-frequency hearing loss were reported by Harris and Glattke [1988]. At high frequencies, DPOAE amplitudes and I/O functions were significantly different when compared to 20 normal subjects. If hearing thresholds at predetermined frequencies were better than 15 dB HL, DPOAE were always detected, and they were absent or attenuated if thresholds exceeded 50 dB HL. Considerable variation was noted in the range between these two threshold values.

Figure 13 shows an example of DPOAE measurement in an asymmetrical high-frequency hearing loss. While the primaries were located in a frequency range with normal hearing thresholds in the right ear and evoked a clear DPOAE, the hearing threshold was elevated above 50 dB in this frequency range at left and no DPOAE could be recorded.

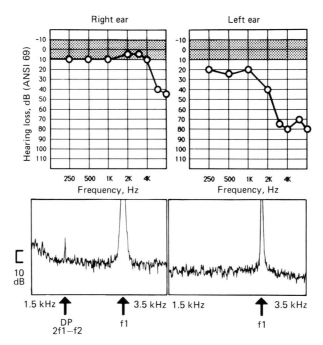

Fig. 13. Example of DPOAE $2f_1 - f_2$ at 2 kHz in an ear with asymmetrical high-frequency hearing loss. $f_1 = 2.857$ kHz, $f_2 = 3.714$ kHz, $f_2/f_1 = 1.3$, $f_1 = f_2 = 70$ dB SPL. The geometric mean of f_1 and f_2 was at 3.257 kHz, showing a hearing threshold of less than 10 dB at right, and over 70 dB at left. A clear emission is evoked at right and no emission is detectable at left.

In conclusion, DPOAE have some promise for clinical applications though their relations to hearing thresholds are not entirely clear. A relatively simple relationship as was seen for TEOAE seems not to be present. An additional difficulty is represented by the multitude of parameters that have to be considered and that can vary. The main advantage of DPOAE testing may lie in the possibility of a relatively frequency-specific measurement of OAE, thereby providing an objective supplement to the pure tone audiogram.

6.4. Findings in Animals

Probably the first DPOAE in animals were reported by Kim et al. [1980] in the cat, Mountain [1980] in the guinea pig, and Siegel et al. [1982] in the chinchilla. Subsequently, robust DPOAE that were relatively easy to record were detected in many common laboratory animals. Additionally, correlations with CM measurements could be demonstrated [Kemp and Brown, 1983a, 1984]. The measurement of DPOAE has been developed into important laboratory methods in hearing research [Horner et al., 1985; Martin et al., 1987a, b; Lonsbury-Martin et al., 1987; Lenoir and Puel, 1987; Brown, 1988]. Table 14 summarizes papers about DPOAE in different species and the DP that were mainly studied. In all these animals, DPOAE were regularly recorded provided that normal hearing with normal middle ear function was assumed.

6.4.1. Amplitude. Contrary to other classes of emissions, DPOAE can be recorded with relatively large amplitudes in many common laboratory animals. Amplitudes of only 30 dB less than the primaries were found mainly in rodents for DP at $2f_1-f_2$. For example, Brown and Kemp [1984] reported a value of 40 dB less than the primaries in the gerbil, and Schmiedt [1986a] and Brown [1987] of 30–40 dB less. Similar values were found in the chinchilla with 30–50 dB less than the primaries [Zurek et al., 1982; Siegel et al., 1982], in the mouse with 20–50 dB [Horner et al., 1985], in the rat at higher frequencies with 30–40 dB [Lenoir and Puel, 1987; Brown, 1987], and in the rabbit with 30–40 dB less [Lonsbury-Martin et al., 1987]. Guinea pigs exhibited a somewhat smaller amplitude of about 40 dB less [Brown, 1987], and cats had even smaller amplitudes of 40–65 dB below the primaries [Schmiedt, 1986a; Wiederhold et al., 1986].

The individual variability reported by the above-mentioned investigators showed a standard deviation of approximately 10 dB. In general, the highest amplitudes were found in frequency ranges with best hearing for the species examined [Horner et al., 1985; Schmiedt, 1986a; Lonsbury-Martin et al., 1987; Brown, 1987]. For example, rats had their highest DPOAE amplitudes at higher frequenceis [Lenoir and Puel, 1987; Brown, 1987] than gerbils or guinea pigs [Brown, 1987]. However, the correlation of DPOAE amplitudes with measures of hearing thresholds such as summating action potentials [Schmiedt, 1986a] was not always straightforward. This probably can be expected, since a number of factors including the multitude of parameters involved, uncertainties about the generation site of DP, and nonmonotonous I/O functions make such comparisons difficult.

The frequency distance between the primaries was an important variable of DPOAE amplitudes. An f_2/f_1 ratio of 1.2–1.3 was found to be most effective in the gerbil [Kemp and Brown, 1984], in the cat [Wiederhold et al., 1986], in the mouse [Horner et al., 1985], and in the rabbit [Lonsbury-Martin et al., 1987]. In addition, primaries with higher frequencies required lower ratios for the generation of maximal DPOAE amplitudes as opposed to those with lower frequencies. The levels of the primaries were also important, in that f_1 amplitudes of about 10 dB louder than f_2 evoked the strongest DPOAE [Brown, 1987]. Thus, many basic features of DPOAE in animals were found to be remarkably similar to those found in human ears.

Table 14. DPOAE reported in animals

Species	DP examined	Authors
Cat	$2f_1-f_2$ f_2-f_1	Kim et al. [1980] Fahey and Allen [1985, 1986] Dolan and Abbas [1985a, b] Wiederhold et al. [1986] Schmiedt [1986a]
Guinea pig	f_2-f_1 sidebands	Mountain [1980] Brown [1987] Brown [1988]
Chinchilla	$2f_1-f_2$ f_2-f_1 $2f_2-f_1$	Siegel et al. [1982] Siegel and Kim [1982a, b] Zurek et al. [1982] Clark et al. [1984]
Gerbil	$2f_1-f_2$ f_2-f_1 3f 4f sidebands	Schmiedt and Adams [1981] Schmiedt and Addy [1982] Brown and Kemp [1983, 1984, 1985] Kemp and Brown [1983a, b, 1984, 1986] Schmiedt [1986a–c] Brown [1987] Brown [1988]
Rabbit	$2f_1-f_2$ $2f_2-f_1$ $3f_1-2f_2$	Martin et al. [1987a, b] Stainbeck et al. [1987] Lonsbury-Martin et al. [1987]
Mouse	$2f_1-f_2$	Horner et al. [1985]
Alligator lizard	$2f_1-f_2$ $2f_2-f_1$	Rosowski et al. [1984b]
Rat	$2f_1-f_2$ sidebands	Lenoir and Puel [1987] Brown [1987]

6.4.2. Input-Output Function. The I/O function of DPOAE in animals generally showed one of two forms, being either more or less linear with a slope of about 1 and a saturation at stimulus levels of about 70 dB SPL, or having nonmonotonous dips at stimulus levels of 60–70 dB SPL. Such I/O functions were reported for the cat [Kim et al., 1980; Wiederhold et al., 1986], chinchilla [Zurek et al., 1982], gerbil [Kemp and Brown, 1983a; Brown, 1987], mouse [Horner et al., 1985], rat [Lenoir and Puel, 1987; Brown, 1987], guinea pig [Brown, 1987], and rabbit [Lonsbury-Martin et al., 1987]. However, the exact shape of the function depended on the particular DP examined, the frequency range of the primaries, and the f_2/f_1 ratio.

The best examined DP is that of the frequency at $2f_1-f_2$. This is the DP with the highest amplitude in the vast majority of conditions and with I/O functions of almost always a slope of 1 at stimulus levels less than 60 dB SPL. Therefore, the 'threshold' of this DPOAE is a function of the noise floor of the measuring system. In common laboratory animals, this threshold can be expected to be at 20–40 dB SPL, assuming a noise floor of about -10 dB SPL and DPOAE amplitudes of 30–40 dB less than the stimulus level.

Nonmonotonous dips were observed more often at higher frequency ranges and with lower f_2/f_1 ratios. At least two different mechanisms are thought to be responsible for the generation of these dips: phase cancellation between two or more acoustic components [Zwicker, 1980a, 1986c; Schmiedt, 1986b; Brown, 1987], and superpostition of two different, level-dependent DP components [Rosowski et al., 1984b; Schmiedt, 1986c; Brown, 1987; Lonsbury-Martin et al., 1987]. Phase cancellation is more likely to appear at low f_2/f_1 ratios and cancellations may occur between primaries or between DP and primaries. With regard to superposition of two components, several lines of evidence suggest that DPOAE consist of a low-level component with linear growth at low stimulus levels and saturation at about 60 dB, and a high-level component with steeper slopes and characteristics of a power series. The superposition of these two components could create dips at stimulus levels of about 60 dB SPL.

The presence of a nonmonotonous I/O function may lead to seemingly paradoxical results if thresholds are varied, e.g. through acoustic overstim-ulation, and if only single level measurements are taken. A rise in threshold such as a TTS may led to a shift of the I/O function to the right, and a dip could thus become a peak. A schematic illustration of such a shift of the I/O function is depicted in figure 14. A rise in DPOAE amplitude could be measured at a single point, although the total amplitude would have been reduced. Therefore, the measurement of complete I/O functions are essential when DPOAE are used to monitor hearing functions.

6.4.3. Latency. The latencies of DPOAE were measured as group latencies when the primaries were swept in frequency [Kemp and Brown, 1983b, 1986; Brown and Kemp, 1985; Kemp, 1986]. Different latencies were found with different conditions. If the primaries were swept with stable and relatively high f_2/f_1 ratios, a short group latency of less than 1 ms was generally measured which did not change significantly with frequency. If, however, the higher-frequency primary was kept at a fixed frequency and only f_1 was swept, longer latencies of 2–5 wavelengths or 1–3 ms were found [Kemp and Brown, 1983a, 1986; Brown and Kemp, 1985]. Latencies changed systematically with different frequencies of f_2 and with changing

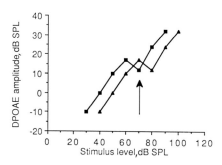

Fig. 14. Schematic illustration of an apparent amplitude increase at a single measuring level (arrow), despite decrease of the total amplitude of DPOAE. This effect occurs through a shift to the right of a nonmonotonous I/O function.

f_2/f_1 ratios. The latency grew longer with lower frequencies of f_2 and with smaller f_2/f_1 ratios. Additionally, Brown and Kemp [1985] found shorter latencies for DPOAE with frequencies higher than the primaries, such as $2f_2-f_1$, compared to those with lower frequencies, such as $2f_1-f_2$.

These findings can be interpreted as a lack of place-fixed emission frequencies in the case of wide and stable f_2/f_1 ratios. When the second primary is kept at a constant frequency, it acts as an induced irregularity of the basilar membrane at a fixed site, thereby leading to the systematic changes of group latencies [Kemp, 1986].

6.4.4. Post-Mortem Properties. The behavior of DPOAE following lethal anoxia or drug overdose initially led to seemingly paradoxical results. While Schmiedt and Adams [1981] found persistent DPOAE with nearly stable amplitudes up to 1 h after death, Kemp and Brown [1984] invariably found amplitude reductions of more than 20 dB 5–10 min after death. Both sets of experiments were conducted in the same species, the gerbil, and with the same DPOAE, $2f_1-f_2$. An explanation of these results was later offered by Schmiedt [1986c], who could demonstrate a dependence of the post-mortem properties of DPOAE on the stimulus level. The amplitude of DPOAE evoked by primary levels of more than 70 dB SPL declined only slowly during the first 2 h postmortem, while those evoked by levels less than 70 dB SPL were reduced to the noise floor within 10–30 min after death. These findings were later confirmed by Lonsbury-Martin et al., [1987] in the rabbit for DPOAE at both $2f_1-f_2$ and $2f_2-f_1$.

Possibly, a second component of DPOAE with different generation mechanisms appears at higher stimulus levels. Further evidence for such a component was already presented in the discussion of I/O functions. Though this component seems to be much more stable to anoxia, several findings suggest that its generation mechanism is still physiologically vulnerable. Particularly interesting is the finding that this component could be fatigued with acoustic overstimulation and, thereafter, showed recovery in animals which were dead for more than 1 h [Lonsbury-Martin et al., 1987]. Additionally, Schmiedt and Adams [1981] demonstrated the complete disappearance of DPOAE after perfusion of the cochlea with solutions of KCl. Findings somewhat in contradiction to such a second component were reported by Horner et al. [1985] in the mouse. They found a reduction of DPOAE amplitudes to the noise floor within 10 min, even with stimulus levels of 90 dB SPL.

6.4.5. Influence of Efferent Stimulation. The relative simplicity of DPOAE measurements in many laboratory animals and their noninvasive characteristics led to the use of DPOAE in studies involving a number of influences on the cochlea including stimulations of the efferent cochlear nerve fibers.

The influence of electrical stimulation of the efferent fibers on DPOAE were reported by Mountain [1980] and Siegel and Kim [1982a, b]. Mountain [1980] found a reduction of the DPOAE amplitude at f_2/f_1 in the guinea pig which was most pronounced at low stimulus levels and reached values of about 70%. Siegel and Kim [1982b] found more complex changes studying the DP at f_2-f_1 and at $2f_1-f_2$ in chinchillas. The DPOAE amplitude could be reduced, enhanced or unchanged during electrical stimulations of the efferent fibers. No systematic relations of these changes to stimulus levels, stimulus frequencies, or to the DP at f_2-f_1 or $2f_1-f_2$ could be demonstrated.

Recent evidence suggests that these findings were obtained under complicating conditions. For example, anesthesia was demonstrated to have a major effect by itself on the DPOAE at f_2-f_1 [Brown, 1988]. This is most likely mediated by efferent innervation. Additionally, the levels of electrical stimulations used in these experiments were probably unphysiological [Kemp and Souter, 1988]. Nevertheless, the findings gave an early indication that the outer hair cells, being the primary cells innervated by the efferent system, are linked to the generation of OAE. More detailed results about the action of efferent innervation were later reported by Guinan [1986] and Kemp and Souter [1988]. However, these investigators used SFOAE and not DPOAE.

6.4.6. Suppression. Suppression tuning curves of DPOAE were mainly studied by Kemp and Brown in gerbils [Brown and Kemp, 1983, 1984; Kemp and Brown, 1984] and Martin et al. [1987a] in rabbits. The shape of these curves was dependent on the parameters of the primaries, such as frequencies, levels, or f_2/f_1 ratios, and on the particular DP frequency.

In general, suppression tuning curves of $2f_1-f_2$ DPOAE were comparable to those found with other OAE classes. Suppression with weakest stimuli was obtained in the frequency range between the two primaries and the DP frequency itself had little influence on the curve [Brown and Kemp, 1984; Martin et al., 1987a]. This implies that the DP $2f_1-f_2$ is generated at a frequency place between the primaries. Since the tip of the suppression curve was shifted from higher to lower frequencies with increasing primary levels, the higher frequency primary may be more important with relatively weak primary levels of about 40 dB SPL [Brown and Kemp, 1984]. However, complex and poorly understood effects may be involved when a third external tone, namely the suppressor, is introduced into the nonlinear interaction between the two primaries, and an exact determination of the DP generation site by suppression measurements alone may not be possible.

Complex and individually varied suppression curves were found at the DP $2f_2-f_1$ [Martin et al., 1987a]. The low frequency slopes of the curves were comparable to those of the DP $2f_1-f_2$. However, maximal suppression was not between the primaries, but at higher frequencies near the DP frequency, suggesting a generation site of this DP at or near the DP frequency. The measurement of the high-frequency slope was difficult because of large, unsystematic amplitude changes with little frequency changes and because of technical limitations.

Essentially the same conclusions as those obtained with suppression concerning the generation site of the two DPOAE at $2f_1-f_2$ and $2f_2-f_1$ could be reached [Martin et al., 1987a] when the frequencies of the primaries were swept around an interfering tone of constant frequency. Using similar methods, Schmiedt [1986b] assumed the generation site of the third harmonic DPOAE of a single tone to be located near the DP frequency and not at the primary frequency.

6.4.7. Noise Exposure. A number of studies examined the influence of acoustic overstimulations on DPOAE. A wide variety of different durations and stimuli were used with the aim of answering very different questions ranging from simulation of chronic noise induced hearing loss [Zurek et al., 1982] to the study of short-term adaptations [Dolan and Abbas, 1985a]. Table 15 summarizes species, exposure levels, durations and frequencies of exposure of such studies reported in the literature. Several of these studies are not directly relevant to the understanding of DPOAE, but all demonstrated the possibilities of DPOAE measurements in hearing research.

Changes of DPOAE induced by acoustic overstimulation can contribute to the understanding of the temporal and place-related properties of these emissions. This is especially true for short exposures that are considered to induce only reversible changes at the hair cell level. Such studies

Table 15. Synopsis of studies using DPOAE in noise exposure

	Species	Level dB SPL	Duration min	Frequency kHz
Kim et al. [1980]	cat	90	2	1.9–2
Zurek et al. [1982]	chinchilla	108	105	4 OBN
		95	360/36 d*	0.5 OBN
Siegel et al. [1982]	chinchilla	108	120	4 OBN
Rosowski et al. [1984b]	alligator lizard	90–110	0.5–120	2
Dolan and Abbas [1985a]	cat	70–90	1	0.5–8
Schmiedt [1986a]	gerbil, cat	85–95	12–12	3.1, 4
Wiederhold et al. [1986]	cat	90–110?	10–60?	0.5, 4, 8
Stainback et al. [1987]	cat	100	60	4
Martin et al. [1987a]	rabbit	90	3	1.4–6.6

OBN = Octave band noise; * 6 h/day for 36 days.

were reported by Kim et al. [1980], Dolan and Abbas [1985a, b], Schmiedt [1986a], and Martin et al. [1987a]. Kim et al. [1980] demonstrated that the time course of DPOAE amplitude recovery was similar to that found in measurements of single nerve fibers. This fact was also noted by others [Dolan and Abbas, 1985; Martin et al., 1987a]. The recovery function was measured with different time resolutions. While Dolan and Abbas [1985a, b] demonstrated a biphasic recovery function for $2f_1-f_2$ using very short exposures and a high time resolution, other investigators [Kim et al., 1980; Martin et al., 1987a] generally considered only a slower acting second component.

Using recovery functions after short exposures, Martin et al. [1987a] were able to confirm the different generation sites of DPOAE at $2f_1-f_2$ and $2f_2-f_1$. These findings were already suggested by findings in suppression experiments mentioned above. Considering the well-known half-octave shift [Hirsh and Bilger, 1955], which has been demonstrated to apply for DPOAE as well [Schmiedt, 1986a], these experiments located the generation site of $2f_1-f_2$ at the frequencies of the primaries, and of $2f_2-f_1$ near the DP frequency. Figure 15 summarizes some of these findings.

The changes of DPOAE after induction of noise-induced hearing loss was also used to correlate changes in DPOAE with those of well established measures of hearing function. For example, Dolan and Abbas [1985a] compared the recovery functions of DPOAE with those of summating action potentials. Besides general similarities of the two recovery functions, the DPOAE amplitude often did not reach its prestimulation level within the examined time frame, in contrast to the potential amplitude. General agreement between the induced changes of summating action potentials

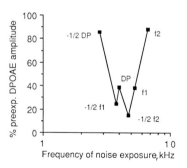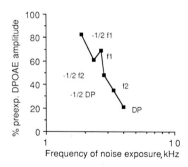

Fig. 15. DPOAE amplitude reduction 10 s after noise exposures of 90 dB SPL and 3 min. The frequency of the exposures were chosen to correspond to the frequency of the primaries or of the DP, and half an octave below these frequencies for compensation of half-octave shifts. Left panel: DPOAE at $2f_1-f_2$; right panel: DPOAE at $2f_2-f_1$. Both DPOAE were at 4 kHz. Maximal reduction, suggesting strongest influence on DPOAE generation, occurred at the primary frequencies in $2f_1-f_2$, and at the DP frequency in $2f_2-f_1$. Redrawn from Martin et al. [1987a], with permission of the publisher.

and DPOAE were found by Schmiedt [1986a] and Wiederhold et al. [1986] though they used quite different parameters. However, Schmiedt [1986a] pointed out that the agreement mainly concerned changes of DPOAE rather than absolute values of DPOAE in dB SPL. Good correlations between changes of behaviorally measured hearing thresholds and DPOAE were reported by Zurek et al. [1982]. In addition, even modest lesions induced by moderate overstimulations of 100 dB SPL for 1 h [Stainback et al., 1987] could be detected as a permanent reduction of DPOAE amplitudes in the corresponding frequency range.

In conclusion, it seems possible to reliably assess noise-induced hearing loss with DPOAE. Histological findings [Zurek et al., 1982; Clark et al., 1984; Stainback et al., 1987] supported this conclusion.

6.4.8. Influence of Drugs. The influence of drugs on DPOAE has been only sporadically examined. Furosemide injections were shown to induce a parallel reduction and subsequent reappearance of DPOAE and CM potentials [Kemp and Brown, 1984], when primaries of less than 70 dB SPL were used. No effect on DPOAE could be found by the administration of aspirin in a monkey [Martin et al., 1988], although SOAE and SFOAE were abolished. Such a dissociation between DPOAE and SOAE has already been mentioned for humans (6.2.5.) [Wier et al., 1988]. Since this monkey showed OAE very similar to those of human ears, the parallel findings are not surprising. Unfortunately, the effect of aspirin on other laboratory animals is not known.

Drugs used for anesthesia may also influence DPOAE, although no consistent and systematic effects have been demonstrated. Lonsbury-Martin et al. [1987] found no changes of DPOAE I/O functions between awake rabbits and those anesthetized with Ketamin and Xylazine when DP at $2f_1-f_2$, $3f_1-f_2$, or $2f_2-f_1$ were examined. Complex changes of f_2-f_1 during anesthesia were reported by Brown [1988] in the guinea pig. The depth of anesthesia seemed to be more important than the particular drugs used. While systematic changes of the f_2-f_1 amplitude during continuous weak acoustic stimulation were found in lightly anesthetized subjects, amplitudes varied widely under deep anesthesia. Since similar changes could be induced by stimulation of the contralateral ear, an influence of the efferent cochlear innervation was suggested. No such changes were seen at the DPOAE $2f_1-f_2$.

6.4.9. Relation to Outer Hair Cells. A number of findings, some of which have been discussed above, suggests that DPOAE are intimately linked to outer hair cell functions. These findings include the demonstration of changes of DPOAE with stimulation of the efferent cochlear fibers and with acoustic overstimulation. Both manipulations are known to primarily effect outer hair cells. In addition, Horner et al. [1985] examined different strains of mice with genetic abnormalities of the hearing system. While normal mice showed DPOAE at $2f_1-f_2$ comparable to those of other rodents, no DPOAE were detected in mutant mice with dysplasia of the whole cochlea or the stria vascularis. Other mutants with central deafness and anatomically normal cochleas exhibited DPOAE with the same properties as those of normal mice. However, in the Bronx waltz mouse, a mutant with a full complement of outer hair cells but only about 20% of inner hair cells, DPOAE with smaller amplitudes and thresholds of about 30 dB higher were found. If these findings are considered alone, they do not support the primary importance of outer hair cells for DPOAE. Explanations for the discrepancy with other evidence include morphological and functional aspects. The rows of outer hair cells in these mice were disrupted and lacked their normal order, making mechanical and/or functional defects probable. Additionally, an intact mechanical and/or electrical connection between inner and outer hair cells could be necessary for the generation of DPOAE.

7. Generation of Otoacoustic Emissions and Clinical Implications

OAE are generated in the cochlea. More precisely, they are generated by the preneural elements of the cochlea between the stapes footplate and the synapses of the afferent cochlear nerve fibers. Important hydromechanical and mechanical events take place in this section of the hearing system as well as the transduction of the signal from mechanical into bioelectrical energy. Whatever the exact mechanism for the generation of OAE may be, it is intimately linked to these events.

7.1. Place- and Wave-Fixed Otoacoustic Emissions

Two different relations of OAE to the basilar membrane can be distinguished [Kemp, 1986]: (1) a place-fixed relationship, and (2) a wave-fixed relationship. Place-fixed emissions show constant frequencies that do not change substantially with different stimuli. The best example may be SOAE with their characteristic frequencies. These constant frequencies are represented by fixed places along the cochlear partition. Several lines of evidence, including anatomical findings [Clark et al., 1984; Lonsbury-Martin et al., 1988b], species differences in hair cell and OAE patterns (sections 3.4, 4.4, 5.3, 6.4), and modeling or theoretical considerations [Sutton and Wilson, 1983; Zwicker, 1986a–c; Lumer, 1987a, b; Furst and Lapid, 1988], suggest that irregularities of the mechanical impedance are present at these places.

Wave-fixed emissions, on the other hand, show frequencies which depend on the stimulus frequency. The most typical examples may be DPOAE with their mathematically defined frequency relations to the stimulus. The 'place' of wave-fixed emissions on the basilar membrane is not fixed; they can occur at any frequency. A preexisting irregularity of basilar membrane impedance that exceeds average variations cannot be assumed at wave-fixed emission frequencies.

The classification in place- and wave-fixed emissions is, first of all, practical in nature. It does not imply, a priori, differences in basic generation mechanisms. The commonly used classification of OAE according to the stimulus type, which was described in section 2.1 and on which the present overview was based, may incorporate within the same class wave- and place-fixed emissions. On the other hand, close relationships exist among these classes of OAE, and the same place-fixed emissions may be evoked by different stimulus presentations. Table 16 tries to relate the two different classifications of OAE to each other.

It is remarkable that the classification in place- and wave-fixed emissions also quite effectively separates the different findings in different species. For one thing, place-fixed emissions are found mainly in human ears and possibly in nonhuman primates, but they are rare or difficult to detect in rodent ears. For another, wave-fixed emissions are readily recorded in rodent ears, and their detection in human ears is more difficult. Presuming that place-fixed emissions are linked to impedance irregularities,

Table 16. Place- and wave-fixed OAE

	Place-fixed	Wave-fixed
No external stimulation	SOAE	–
Transient stimulation	TEOAE (narrowband)	TEOAE (broadband?)
Low-level sinusoid	SFOAE (long latency)	SFOAE (short latency)
Medium-level sinuoids	DPOAE modulations ($f_2/f_1 < \approx 1.25$)	DPOAE ($f_2/f_1 > \approx 1.25$)

it follows that the human cochlea must have a less regular impedance structure along the basilar membrane than, for example, the rodent cochlea. Primates must have impedance structures closer to the human than to rodent cochleas. The same may be true for the bat cochlea in regions were ultrasound is detected.

The following discussion provides more details and implications which can be drawn from table 16 for the different classes of OAE.

7.1.1. Implications for Spontaneous Emissions. The biological and clinical significance of SOAE is not entirely clear at the moment. The most pertinent question from a clinical point of view concerns their possible connection to subtle pathological changes within the cochlea. Spontaneous emissions are always place-fixed emissions, and a localized pathological change along the basilar membrane may be responsible for the impedance irregularity involved in the emission generation.

Indeed, some experimental and circumstantial evidence suggests such a possibility. Since SOAE can be detected in only about a third of seemingly healthy ears, they are clearly not invariably associated with normal cochlear function. Moreover, anecdotal case reports linked the appearance of SOAE to acoustic overstimulations [Flottorp, 1953; Wilson and Sutton, 1981; Norton and Mott, 1987; Rebillard et al., 1987]. Experimental evidence for an association of noise trauma and SOAE was presented by Clark et al. [1984] in chinchillas, including histopathological findings in the cochlea. However, these SOAE in many details resembled the rare high-level emissions of human ears (section 3.3.1) and not the commonly found SOAE. High-level SOAE seem to be associated with special circumstances, and they may well be an expression of some functional abnormalities within the cochlea.

However, other evidence suggests that the generation of SOAE is possible within normally structured cochleas. First of all, SOAE are found only in frequency ranges where hearing threshold is normal or near normal. While this finding alone does not exclude subtle pathological changes at a limited number of hair cells, taken together with the same or even higher incidence of SOAE in babies and small children [Strickland et al., 1985] and the significant higher bilateral incidence in individuals with SOAE, it strongly contradicts acquired pathological changes as a reason for SOAE. Moreover, structural features that are already present at birth and that are associated with normal hearing thresholds can hardly be called pathological. Anatomical findings [Lonsbury-Martin et al., 1988b] in a rhesus monkey with place-fixed emissions, which were very similar to those commonly found in humans, pointed to specific patterns of outer hair cells as the generation site of SOAE. Besides general irregularities of the hair cell pattern, a fourth row of outer hair cells appeared in intervals along the organ of Corti (fig. 4). These irregularities were mainly found in the apical portions of the cochlea and the intervals correlated with the frequency spacing of place-fixed emissions.

Such irregular hair cell patterns could lead to impedance irregularities responsible for place-fixed emissions. They are commonly found in cochleas of humans [Engström et al., 1966; Bredberg, 1968] and rhesus monkeys [Hawkins et al., 1985; Lonsbury-Martin et al., 1988b]. However, SOAE are generally detected in only a minority of normal ears. Theoretically [Kemp, 1986; Zwicker, 1986b; Lumer, 1987a], the sporadic occurrence of SOAE could be explained within the normal function of the cochlea when special conditions are met.

Nevertheless, missing hair cells could create such conditions as well, and 'pathological' SOAE could coexist with 'normal' SOAE. This uncertainty cannot be resolved at the moment, since no distinctions between these two theoretical forms of SOAE are known. Possibly, patterns of place-fixed emissions recorded during influences damaging the cochlea could help to differentiate place-fixed emissions due to irregularities of hair cell patterns that are genetically present from those that are induced by pathology.

7.1.2. Implications for Transiently Evoked Emissions. The arguments and questions about SOAE from the foregoing could be applied, in principle, to each form of place-fixed emissions. Since the majority of TEOAE in man are typical place-fixed emissions, the question of pathological or physiological origin could also be applied to TEOAE. However, the assumption of a sole pathological basis becomes unlikely in human TEOAE, since these emissions can be detected in nearly all normal hearing ears. A combination of pathological and physiological causes is conceivable but, similar to what has already been said, this hypothesis is not easily tested and, for the moment, unresolved.

Besides constant emission frequencies, corresponding to place-fixed emissions, TEOAE show a second, broadly tuned emission component with frequencies that most probably depend on the stimulus frequencies [Probst et al., 1986; Norton and Neely, 1987; Bonfils et al., 1988a]. This broadband component would fulfil the main conditions for wave-fixed emissions: It can be generated along a continuous frequency range at any place and its frequency spectrum corresponds to the stimulus spectrum. Such a wave-fixed component of TEOAE may be regularly present in human ears [Norton and Neely, 1987; Bonfils et al., 1988a]. However, its detection seems to be difficult for a number of reasons. Most important, the amplitude of this component is probably quite small and, in most ears, prominent place-fixed emissions may interfere with it. Additionally, the latency of this component is not clear, but it may be considerably shorter than those of place-fixed emissions and, therefore, interfere with the stimulus ringing. Though this component may be a means of frequency-specfic testing with TEOAE, practical experience did not show its clinical usefulness [Probst et al., 1986; Lutman and Fleming, 1988]. For the moment, TEOAE must be considered in a clinical setting to test essentially place-fixed emissions. Therefore, they primarily provide information about fixed, idiosyncratic frequencies with wide variations in numbers and places from ear to ear. However, since nearly all human ears exhibit some emission frequencies between 1–2 kHz, TEOAE may be an ideal means for screening.

It is conceivable that quantitative differences of impedance changes are responsible for the different components and that there is a smooth transition between them. Relatively small impedance changes must be assumed along any 'normal' cochlear partition which may lead to wave-fixed emissions. Localized, more prominent irregularities could induce a wide range of quantitatively different impedance changes leading to evoked emission frequencies with different damping. Lack of damping would induce spontaneous oscillations or SOAE. Several findings support such a hypothesis [Wit et al., 1981; Rutten and Buisman, 1983; Probst et al., 1986; Zwicker, 1986a, b; Norton and Neely, 1987].

7.1.3. Implications for Stimulus-Frequency Emissions. Analogous implications to those for place-fixed TEOAE are valid for human SFOAE. However, a SFOAE-component with wave-fixed characteristics has not been convincingly demonstrated in human ears, in contrast to several laboratory animals [Kemp and Brown, 1983a, b; Rosowski et al., 1984a;

Kemp and Souter, 1988]. Thus, SFOAE can clearly represent both place- and wave-fixed emissions, although in different species. The typical properties of place-fixed SFOAE, such as those found in human ears, are relatively large amplitudes at low stimulus levels, saturation at higher levels, and a relatively long group latency. Since the group latency is dependent on a change of phase between stimulus and emission [Kemp, 1986], a long latency should be expected when the stimulus frequency is swept and the emission is generated at a fixed place along the basilar membrane. In contrast, a short latency occurs when the stimulus frequency and the emission place are simultaneously changing, i.e. when a wave-fixed emission is present. As a matter of fact, such short latencies were demonstrated in SFOAE of gerbils [Kemp and Brown, 1983a]. Additionally, wave-fixed SFOAE may have a component at higher stimulus levels that does not show saturation, and they may be difficult to detect at low levels.

For clinical purposes, much the same conclusions may be valid for SFOAE as for TEOAE. However, the clinical assessment of SFOAE is not yet done.

7.1.4. Implications for Distortion Product Emissions. The frequency of DPOAE is determined by the stimulus frequencies. Therefore, DPOAE cannot be generated by place-fixed mechanisms and they represent typical examples of wave-fixed emissions. Presumably, the irregularity leading to DPOAE is created by the stimulus-induced travelling wave [Kemp, 1986]. The properties of DPOAE would then depend on stimulus parameters such as primary levels and f_2/f_1 ratio. For example, a relatively high group latency of DPOAE was found when only f_1 was swept and f_2 was kept at a constant frequency acting like a place-fixed emission [Kemp, 1986]. If, however, frequency sweeps with a constant f_2/f_1 ratio were examined, the latency was dependent on the value of the ratio. Distortion product emissions evoked with a relatively high f_2/f_1 ratio of 1.3 showed short latencies in both humans and gerbils [Kemp, 1986]. In cochleas with place-fixed emissions, the influence of these emissions on DPOAE was most prominent when small f_2/f_1 ratio and relatively low stimulus levels were used. The use of such parameters leads to modulations of DPOAE amplitudes which become largest at frequencies of place-fixed emissions. Such modulations have been shown repeatedly in human ears [Wilson, 1980d; Wit et al., 1981; Kemp, 1986; Wier et al., 1988; Furst et al., 1988], and they are generally lacking in rodent ears. Moreover, the average amplitudes of DPOAE are much smaller in ears with place-fixed emissions than in ears showing mainly wave-fixed emissions. Such differences were predicted in models [Furst and Lapid, 1988] for cochleas with different structural uniformity along the cochlear partition. Regular structures, implying smoothly changing impedance along the basilar membrane, were shown in this model to generate large DPOAE amplitudes but no place-fixed emissions. Therefore, the regular hair cell patterns normally found in ears of common laboratory animals, such as rodents or rabbits, may provide a possible explanation of their higher amplitude DPOAE.

For clinical purposes, a frequency-specific testing of OAE not dependent on the idiosyncratic frequencies of place-fixed emissions would be desirable. It could offer an objective counterpart to the clinically important pure tone audiogram. Wave-fixed emissions in general, and DPOAE in particular, can be considered for such testing. Preliminary findings of Kemp et al. [1986], Lonsbury-Martin et al. [1988a] and of our own laboratory [Probst et al., 1989] indicate the feasibility of such tests. However, many problems related to parametric or technical details are not sufficiently examined to draw final conclusions. In addition, DPOAE do not test pure tones but, at best, localized frequency regions since at least two frequencies of the primaries are involved.

7.2. Generation Mechanisms

7.2.1. Basic Mechanisms. OAE are acoustic signals that are generated, as a final step, by vibrations of the tympanic membrane. This, in turn, is induced by movements of the stapes footplate. Therefore, a retrograde hydromechanical traveling wave has to be generated within the cochlea.

Though Wilson [1980c] and Wilson and Sutton [1981] first considered the generation of stapes vibrations without traveling waves, which were supposed to occur by volume changes of outer hair cells alone, they abandoned this concept [Wilson and Sutton, 1983] in light of newer measurements of basilar membrane tuning [Sellik et al., 1982; Khanna and Leonard, 1982] and the findings of high-level SOAE. All the same, volume or, rather, length changes of outer hair cells may have essential functions during the generation of OAE [Brownell et al., 1985; Zenner et al., 1987].

At least two fundamentally different possibilities of how a retrograde traveling wave could be generated are conceivable: either by active oscillations at localized places of the basilar membrane, or by reflection of an anterograde traveling wave within the cochlea. Moreover, the reflection could be passive only, like an acoustic echo, or it could be combined with oscillations at the reflection place, either spontaneously present or induced through the anterograde traveling wave for a limited time period. The passive damping properties of the cochlear mechanical system, such as present post mortem, is reduced by active processes in the physiologically working system. Quantitative changes alone of such an active system may be sufficient for the occurrence of self-oscillations within the cochlea.

Both a reduction of damping or a true amplification of the vibration amplitude require mechanisms that increase the cochlear resonance actively, i.e. that depend on normal metabolism. Positive feedback loops are generally considered necessary for such active systems [Zwicker, 1979a, 1986a; Davis, 1983; Neely and Kim, 1986]. Gold and Pumphrey [1948] and Gold [1948] were probably the first to propose such feedback systems responsible for increasing the frequency resolution of the cochlea. Gold [1948] also predicted the occurrence of spontaneous oscillations and of OAE within such a system. Furthermore, he considered as necessary a saturation of these feedback loops at relatively low levels, since the system would otherwise become instable.

Since the functional details of cochlear resonant systems and its feedback loops are not known, the basic mechanism generating OAE are also not known. Feedback loops could be mechanical [Zwislocki, 1984, 1985] or electromechanical [Weiss, 1982; Mountain et al., 1983; Hubbard and Mountain, 1983; Mountain, 1986]. The transduction process is thought to be reversible, and positive feedback loops could be generated in such a system with appropriate phase relations. The motility of outer hair cells [Brownell et al., 1985], which is capable of high-frequency movements [Zenner et al., 1987], may be the mechanical effector of the amplifying system.

Nonuniformities of the damping factor along the cochlear partition could well be associated with nonuniformities of the mechanical impedance. This is the most likely cause of traveling wave reflections [Sutton and Wilson, 1983; Zwicker, 1986a–c; Lumer 1987a, b; Furst and Lapid, 1988]. A structural basis of such impedance irregularities is generally assumed for place-fixed emissions, whereas nonlinear mechanical disturbances induced by the anterograde traveling wave along the basilar membrane are supposed to be the reflection place for wave-fixed emissions.

7.2.2. Place-Fixed Emissions. Theoretical considerations [Kemp, 1980; Boer, 1983; Boer et al., 1986] and experiments with models [Zwicker, 1986b; Lumer, 1987a; Furst and Lapid, 1988] indicate that localized nonuniformities of the impedance along the cochlear partition are necessary for induction of place-fixed emissions. The degree of local impedance changes and the amount of local resonant amplification determine if place-fixed emissions are generated or not. A reflection of the traveling wave without local amplification would have a loss of energy of about 35 dB according to one calculation [Boer, 1983; Boer et al., 1986]. However, OAE reaching values of 100% returned energy make active systems very likely. Given the incidence and the amplitude of place-fixed emissions in human ears, it can be assumed that the human cochlea is working with more nonuniformities and/or higher amplification factors than, for example, the rodent cochlea.

The finding of SOAE in human ears makes it probable that a true amplification process takes place, and that these are not only reflections. However, these emissions are not, by themselves, proof for an active amplification system exceeding passive damping factors. Theoretically [Kemp, 1981; Bialek, 1983], SOAE could be generated by the combination of multiple reflections and narrow filtering of background noise. Final proof of the true oscillatory nature of SOAE was established by the demonstration of bimodal distributions in amplitude histograms of SOAE [Bialek and Wit, 1984; Wit, 1986]. However, it is an unresolved question if these true oscillations occur within normal functions or only under subtle pathological conditions. The evidence against a hypothesis of sole pathological causes was already discussed (section 7.1.1).

According to the reflection theory of Kemp [1979a, 1980, 1981], acoustic stimulation induces oscillations of the basilar membrane at sites of place-fixed emissions, which are not spontaneously oscillating. These induced oscillations decrease with various time constants, and they generate a retrograde traveling wave that transmits vibrations to the stapes footplate. Additionally, the regrograde traveling wave is again reflected in an apical direction at this point. Depending on the degree of amplification, interfering standing wave patterns of different stabilities may be generated by these multiple reflections and several resonances could appear that would not necessarily correspond to structural irregularities of the cochlear partition. A regular frequency pattern of such emissions has to be assumed. However, such results were only partially found in psychoacoustical measures [Kemp, 1979b], in TEOAE [Kemp and Chum, 1980b], or in SFOAE [Kemp and Chum, 1980a; Zwicker and Schloth, 1984]. Additional supporting evidence for standing wave patterns could be concluded from the increase of the average frequency distances between TEOAE, SFOAE, and SOAE with increasing frequencies [Schloth, 1982; Zwicker and Schloth, 1984; Dallmayr, 1985, 1987].

However, place-fixed emissions are generally found as complex patterns with unique numbers and frequencies in each ear, and it is difficult to explain these patterns with standing waves alone. Several nonuniformities along the cochlear partition must be assumed, each of which may lead to multiple reflections of the traveling wave. Thus, the generation of complex patterns is conceivable. The most likely structural bases of mechanical discontinuities along the cochlear partition are variabilities in the arrangements of outer hair cells and of their connections to the tectorial membrane through the stereocilia. Irregularities of the hair cell pattern can be genetically determined. This may occur either as missing or additional hair cells or through irregular arrangements of a normal complement of hair cells alone. Alternatively, they can be acquired through the loss of hair cells within a regular pattern. Some evidence suggests that genetic patterns may be important in the generation of place-fixed emissions. Manley [1983] pointed out that OAE occur mainly in the apical segments of the cochlea, where the narrower coiling of the cochlea leads to more irregular hair cell patterns during development. Additionally, such irregularities tend to appear in more or less regular intervals along the basilar membrane. This could provide an explanation for the approximate regularity of distances between place-fixed emissions mentioned above [Kemp, 1979b; Kemp and Chum, 1980a, b; Zwicker and Schloth, 1984]. Histological findings in agreement with such a hypothesis were found in a rhesus monkey with human-like OAE [Lonsbury-Martin et al., 1988b]. Parallels between the SFOAE pattern and the pattern of occurrence of a fourth row of outer hair cells were indicative for some connections between the two phenomena. Additional and indirect evidence for a genetic structural basis of irregularities is provided by the high correlation of TEOAE patterns between the ears of individuals, the higher binaural incidence of SOAE, and the same or even higher incidence of place-fixed emissions in newborns and babies. Nonuniform patterns of outer hair cells alone are not sufficient for the generation of place-fixed emissions [Lonsbury-Martin et al., 1988b]. Other conditions must be met that are not known and are probably connected to the basic, unknown mechanism generating OAE.

In conclusion, place-fixed emissions are generated either by localized, spontaneous oscillations or by a combination of traveling wave reflections and evoked, damped oscillations. Spontaneous oscillations induce a retrograde traveling wave and SOAE. The exact generation mechanisms of the spontaneous oscillations are not known but they are thought to be linked to a resonant amplifying system within the organ of Corti. This system most probably includes positive feedback loops, and the mechanical effector may be the outer hair cells. Acoustic stimulation phase-locks such spontaneous oscillations. However, time-limited oscillations with various damping factors can also be evoked at other places along the cochlear partition and, moreover, a reflection of the traveling wave occurs at these places. Structurally, such places probably correspond to nonuniformities in the pattern of outer hair cells. Unique and unknown conditions must be fulfilled for the generation of emissions at such places, since not all irregularities lead to place-fixed emissions. Additionally, interactions among antero- and retrograde traveling waves may also influence the phenomenology of place-fixed emissions.

7.2.3. Wave-Fixed Emissions. In a cochlea with smoothly changing impedance along the basilar membrane, no reflection of a low or medium amplitude traveling wave should occur and no place-fixed emissions should be generated. However, the traveling wave itself can create enough nonuniformity along the cochlear partition for the generation of OAE. The basic mechanism generating such OAE could well be the same as for place-fixed emissions.

The cochlea can be modeled as rows of resonant elements which incorporate nonlinear, amplifying processes [Kim, 1986a, b; Neely and Kim, 1986; Zwicker, 1986a, b; Lumer, 1987a; Furst and Lapid, 1988]. In such models, the smoothness of impedance changes and, thereby, the occurrence of place-fixed OAE is partially determined by the number of elements per distance and the degree of amplification within the elements. Distortion products, however, are thought to be produced within the nonlinear processes of each element. Therefore, nonuniformity is not a necessary condition for the generation of these emissions and DP amplitude is mainly dependent on stimulus parameters.

It is likely that the cochlear system is working physiologically with high amplifications [Kemp, 1988] and that wave-fixed emissions signify normal function of nonlinear, fast-acting processes providing this amplification. Single tones may induce harmonic distortions or, at least in the gerbil, SFOAE representing systematic energy leakage at the stimulus frequency [Kemp, 1986]. For human ears, such an emission component is difficult to detect. On the other hand, transient stimuli with broad frequency spectra should evoke the same amplifying processes, but emissions are difficult to detect in relatively uniform cochleas with this type of stimulation. This may be explained by short latencies and/or internal cancellations within the broad frequency band. The presence of a broadband component in TEOAE of human ears [Probst et al., 1986; Norton and Neely, 1987; Bonfils et al., 1988a] may signify less perfect cancellation, possibly because of relatively weak nonuniformities that are distributed along whole sections of the cochlear partition. This broadband component could, therefore, represent a transition between wave- and place-fixed mechanisms of OAE generation.

Two-tone stimulation leads to interactions between the two traveling waves creating a multitude of DP. The DP $2f_1-f_2$ has been shown to be generated in the frequency range of the primaries [Brown and Kemp, 1984; Martin et al., 1987a], the exact place most likely being the point of maximal interactions between the two traveling waves [Kemp, 1986; Zwicker, 1986c; Martin et al., 1987a]. From the site of generation, the DP is propagated to its apical characteristics frequency place where, for example, it can be percepted psychoacoustically. In addition, interactions with place-fixed emission generators seem to occur also at the characteristic frequency place [Kemp, 1979a; Wilson, 1980d; Wit et al., 1981; Wier et al., 1988], which can lead to modulations of DPOAE. A second propagation from the site of DP generation occurs in a retrograde fashion leading directly to DPOAE [Kemp, 1986; Zwicker, 1986c; Martin et al., 1987a].

Distortion products with frequencies other than $2f_1-f_2$ may be generated at different sites. For example, it was shown [Brown and Kemp, 1985; Martin et al., 1987a] that the DP $2f_2-f_1$ is generated at or basal to its characteristic frequency place. This is basal of the primary frequencies. Therefore, a common generation site for all DP cannot be assumed, although a common generation mechanism is not excluded. It is conceivable, especially at higher stimulus levels, that complicated interactions between the primaries themselves, between DP and the primaries [Matthews and Molnar, 1986], and between different DP can lead to the generation of DP at multiple sites through the same mechanism. In addition, different level-dependent mechanisms are also not excluded. On the contrary, a number of findings suggesting two different mechanisms were reported, including two components of the I/O functions [Rosowski et al., 1984b] and level-dependent differences of DPOAE postmortem [Schmiedt, 1986a; Lonsbury-Martin et al., 1987]. The exact meaning of these results is poorly understood at the moment.

The final phenomenology of DPOAE, as recorded in the ear canal, has to be regarded as a summed vibrational activity of multiple, highly complex interactions at the base of the cochlea [Gibian and Kim, 1982; Brown and Kemp, 1985]. In addition, middle ear transmission may also contribute to these interactions [Dolan and Abbas, 1985a]. Therefore, the 'picture' of DPOAE in the ear canal is not necessarily the same as the picture of DP along the cochlea itself. A perfect agreement of psychoacoustical measurements and OAE measurements cannot be expected and was, in fact, not found [Wilson, 1980d].

In contrast to place-fixed emissions, there is general agreement that wave-fixed emissions are a sign of normal cochlear function. Though the basic mechanism may be the same for place- and wave-fixed emissions, no special conditions have to be met for the generation of wave-fixed emissions. No structural or functional peculiarities are necessary. The physiological amplifying system, presumably including positive feedback loops and the outer hair cells as a mechanical effector, is producing DP at different frequencies and different sites. These DP are partially transmitted to the base of the cochlea where they generate stapes vibrations and DPOAE. From a clinical point of view, DPOAE may offer two distinct advantages. First, DPOAE are produced under normal working conditions of the cochlea and indicate normal function of the outer hair cells. Their demonstration may, therefore, indicate a healthy cochlea. Second, they may offer frequency specificity in OAE testing. However, further investigations will be required to assess the significance of wave-fixed emissions in clinical practice.

7.3. Biological Significance of Otoacoustic Emissions

Are there any specific biological benefits of OAE? Obviously, this question should not be brought forward in this way, as is true for any question about the benefit of isolated biological phenomena. However, in view of the widespread appearance of OAE in different hearing systems, an evolutionary advantage of OAE has to be assumed.

Only SOAE occur in isolation, all other types of OAE appear in conjunction with acoustic stimulations. Since SOAE are exceptional in most species, and since they are not perceived under normal conditions even in humans, it can be assumed that SOAE by themselves do not contribute to the normal processing of acoustic information. Therefore, it can be further assumed that OAE are essentially epiphenomena of some basic hearing mechanism. As a matter of fact, they must be regarded as a by-product of evolutionary improvements of the frequency analyzing capacity and sensitivity of the hearing system.

Two major factors limiting the processing of acoustic information in the mammalian cochlea are rate limitations of the nerve fibers and background noise. These limitations are overcome by frequency analysis and averaging processes [Lewis, 1987]. Both of these are provided by cochlear mechanics. However, the sensitivity found in many hearing systems can only be reached with the help of biological amplification of the acoustic signal. Due to the extraordinary sensitivity of these amplifying processes, which are working at physical limits [Bialek, 1983], and because of their inherent nonlinearities, 'noise' in the form of self-oscillations and distortions occurs. Thus, OAE can be regarded as an evolutionary compromise: In frequency ranges of special interest for an organism, such as those of speech in humans or those of ultrasound orientation calls in bats, the 'price' of self-oscillations is payed for an increase in sensitivity which reaches the limits of what is physically possible. Additionally, nonlinear limitations of the amplification are necessary for reasons of stability, dynamic range, and temporal resolution. An adaptive filter strategy [Lewis, 1987] is used to reach these goals, trading temporal resolution against sensitivity at low signal levels, and frequency resolution against dynamic range and good temporal resolution at higher levels. Again, the 'price' is distortion in the nonlinear processes. However, evolution has incorporated these 'noises' within the hearing system without notable interference of the information processing capability.

The biological significance of OAE are, therefore, not related to the emissions themselves but to their role in helping to understand the underlying mechanisms of the cochlea. The significance of OAE for hearing research lies in the fact that these mechanisms and their functions have mainly been recognized through the detection of OAE. Finally, the clinical significance of OAE comes from the possibility to examine and monitor these cochlear mechanisms in a noninvasive way. The importance and implications of these mechanisms for clinical otology have only begun to be understood.

References

Allen, J.B.: Cochlear modeling. IEEE ASSP Mag. *January:* 3–29 (1985).

Anderson, S.D.: Some ECMR properties in relation to other signals from the auditory periphery. Hear. Res. *2:* 273–296 (1980).

Anderson, S.D.; Kemp D.T.: The evoked cochlear mechanical response in laboratory primates. Archs Oto-Rhino-Lar. *224:* 47–54 (1979).

Antonelli, A.; Grandori, F.: Long-term stability, influence of the head position and modelling considerations for evoked otoacoustic emissions. Scand. Audiol. *25:* suppl., pp. 97–108 (1986).

Bargones, J.Y.; Burns, E.M.: Suppression tuning for spontaneous otoacoustic emissions in infants and adults. J. acoust. Soc. Am. *83:* 1809–1816 (1988).

Beck, D.; Probst, R.: Das Verhalten der spontanen otoakustischen Emissionen unter Narkosebedingungen. Akt. Probl. Otorhinolar. *11:* 313–318 (1988).

Békésy, G. von: Über die nichtlinearen Verzerrungen des Ohres. Ann. phys. Lpz. *20:* 809–811 (1934).

Bialek, W.: Thermal noise and active process in the inner ear: relating theory to experiment; in Klinke, Hartmann, Hearing – physiological bases and psychophysic, pp. 51–57 (Springer, Berlin 1983).

Bialek, W.; Wit, H.P.: Quantum limits to oscillator stability: theory and experiments on acoustic emissions from the human ear. Phys. Lett. *104A:* 173–178 (1984).

Boer, E. de: No sharpening? A challenge for cochlear mechanics. J. acoust. Soc. Am. *73:* 567–573 (1983).

Boer, E. de; Kaernbach, C.; König, P.; Schillen, T.: Forward and reverse waves in the one-dimensional model of the cochlea. Hear. Res. *23:* 1–7 (1986).

Bohne, B.A.; Clark, W.W.: Growth of hearing loss and cochlear lesion with increasing duration of noise exposure; in Hamernik, Henderson, Salvi, New perspectives on noise-induced hearing loss, pp. 283–300 (Raven Press, New York 1982).

Bonfils, P.; Bertrand, Y.; Uziel, A.: Evoked otoacoustic emissions: normative data and presbyacusis. Audiology *27:* 27–35 (1988a).

Bonfils, P.; Piron, J.-P.; Uziel, A.; Pujol, R.: A correlative study of evoked otoacoustic emission properties and audiometric thresholds. Archs Oto-Rhino-Lar. *244:* 53–56 (1988b).

Bonfils, P.; Uziel, A.: Recrutement et diplacousie – conception physiopathologique actuelle. Annls Oto-lar. *104:* 213–217 (1987).

Bonfils, P.; Uziel, A.; Narcy, P.: Apport des émission acoustiques cochléaires en audiologie pédiatrique. Annls Oto-lar. *105:* 109–113 (1988c).

Bonfils, P.; Uziel, A.; Pujol, R.: Evoked oto-acoustic emissions from adults and infants: clinical applications. Acta oto-lar. *105:* 445–449 (1988d).

Bonfils, P.; Uziel, A.; Pujol, R.: Evoked otoacoustic emissions: a fundamental and clinical survey. ORL *50:* 212–218 (1988e).

Bray, P.; Kemp, D.: An advanced cochlear echo technique suitable for infant screening. Br. J. Audiol. *21:* 191–204 (1987).

Bredberg, G.: Cellular patterns and nerve supply of the human organ of Corti. Acta oto-lar. suppl. 236, pp. 1–135 (1968).

Bright, K.E.; Glattke, T.J.: Spontaneous otoacoustic emissions in normal listeners. Am. Sp. Lang. Hear. Ass. *26:* 147 (1984).

Brown, A.M.: Acoustic distortion from rodent ears: a comparison of responses from rats, guinea pigs and gerbils. Hear. Res. *31:* 25–38 (1987).

Brown, A.M.: Continuous low level sound alters cochlear mechanics: an efferent effect? Hear. Res. *34:* 27–38 (1988).

Brown, A.M.; Kemp, D.T.: Otoacoustic emissions: the isosuppression tuning properties of the distortion product $2f_1–f_2$ in gerbil and man. Br. J. Audiol. *17:* 123–124 (1983).

Brown, A.M.; Kemp, D.T.: Suppressibility of the $2f_1–f_2$ stimulated acoustic emissions in gerbil and man. Hear. Res. *13:* 29–37 (1984).

Brown, A.M.; Kemp, D.T.: Intermodulation distortion in the cochlea: could basal vibration be the major cause of round window CM distortion? Hear. Res. *19:* 191–198 (1985).

Brownell, W.E.; Bader, C.R.; Bertrand, D.; Ribaupierre, Y. de: Evoked mechanical responses of isolated cochlear outer hair cells. Science *227:* 194–196 (1985).

Burns, E.M.; Strickland, E.A.; Jones, K.; Tubis, A.: The relationship of threshold fine structure to spontaneous otoacoustic emissions. J. acoust. Soc. Am. *75:* suppl. 1, p. S82 (1984a).

Burns, E.M.; Strickland, E.A.; Tubis, A.; Jones, K.: Interactions among spontaneous emissions. I. Distortion products and linked emissions. Hear. Res. *16:* 271–278 (1984b).

Champlin, C.A.; Norton, S.J.: The effect of intense pure tones on different spontaneous otoacoustic emissions in the same ear. Abstr. 10th Midwinter Research Meet. Ass. Res. Otolaryngol., 1987, p. 20.

Cianfrone, G.; Mattia, M.: Spontaneous otoacoustic emissions from normal human ears preliminary report. Scand. Audiol. *25:* suppl., pp. 121–127.

Citron L.: Observation on a case objective tinnitus. Excerpta Med. Int. Congr. Ser., No. 189, p. 91 (1969).

Clark, W.W.; Kim, D.O.; Zurek, P.M.; Bohne, B.A.: Spontaneous otoacoustic emissions in chinchilla ear canals: correlation with histopathology and suppression by external tones. Hear. Res. *16:* 299–314 (1984).

Collet, L.; Morgon, A.: Oto-acoustic emission and sensorineural hearing loss. Abstr. Int. Symp. Clinical Applications of Otoacoustic Emissions, Montpellier 1988.

Dallmayr, C.: Spontane oto-akustische Emissionen: Statistik und Reaktion auf akustische Störtöne. Acustica *59:* 67–75 (1985).

Dallmayr, C.: Stationary and dynamic properties of simultaneous evoked otoacoustic emissions (SEOAE). Acustica *63:* 243–255 (1987).

Dallos, P.: The role of outer hair cells in cochlear function; in Correia, Perachio, Contemporary sensory neurobiology, pp. 207–230 (Liss, New York 1985).

Davis, H.: An active process in cochlear mechanics. Hear. Res. *9:* 79–90 (1983).

Dear, S.P.; Surrow, J.B.; Schwartz, D.M.; Pribitkin, E.; Saunders, J.C.: Wideband noise exposure augments the amplitude of spontaneous otoacoustic emissions. Abstr. 9th Midwinter Research Meet. Ass. Res. Otolaryngol., 1986, p. 154.

Decker, T.N.; Fritsch, J.H.: Objective tinnitus in the dog. J. Am. Vet. Med. Ass. *180:* 74 (1982).

Dijk, P. van; Wit, H.P.: The occurrence of click-evoked otoacoustic emissions (Kemp echoes) in normal-hearing ears. Scand. Audiol. *16:* 62–64 (1987).

Divenyi, P.L.: Frequency selectivity of the active cochlear filters inferred from otoacoustic emissions evoked by steady-state tones. J. acoust. Soc. Am. *80:* suppl. 1, p. S49 (1986).

Dolan, T.G.; Abbas, P.J.: Changes in the $2f_1-f_2$ acoustic emission and whole-nerve response following sound exposure: long-term effects. J. acoust. Soc. Am. *77:* 1475–1483 (1985a).

Dolan, T.G.; Abbas, P.J.: Short-term effects of sound exposure on the $2f_1-f_2$ acoustic emission. J. acoust. Soc. Am. *77:* 1614–1616 (1985b).

Eggermont, J.: Narrow band AP latencies in normal and recruiting human ears. J. acoust. Soc. Am. *65:* 463–470 (1979).

Elberling, C.; Parbo, J.; Johnsen, N.J.; Bagi, P.: Evoked acoustic emissions: clinical application. Acta oto-lar. suppl. 421, pp. 77–85 (1985).

Engström, H.; Ades, H.W.; Andersson, A.: Structural pattern of the organ of Corti (Williams & Wilkins, Baltimore 1966).

Evans, E.F.; Wilson J.P.; Borerwe, T.A.: Animal models of tinnitus; in Evered, Lawrenson, Tinnitus. Ciba Fdn Symp., pp. 108–138 (Pitman, London 1981).

Fahey, P.F.; Allen, J.B.: Nonlinear phenomena as observed in the ear canal and at the auditory nerve. J. acoust. Soc. Am. *77:* 599–612 (1985).

Fahey, P.F.; Allen, J.B.: Characterization of cubic intermodulation distortion products in the cat external auditory meatus; in Allen, Hall, Hubbard, Neely, Tubis, Peripheral Auditory Mechanisms, pp. 314–321 (Springer, Berlin 1986).

Flottorp, G.: Pure-tone tinnitus evoked by acoustic stimulation: the idiophonic effect. Acta oto-lar. *43:* 396–415 (1953).

Franklin, D.J.; Harris, F.P.; Hawkins, M.D.; Martin, G.K.; Lonsbury-Martin, B.L.: Clinical applications of tests of acoustic distortion products. Abstr. Int. Symp. Clinical Applications of Otoacoustic Emissions, Montpellier 1988.

Frick, L.R.; Matthies, M.L.: Effects of external stimuli on spontaneous otoacoustic emissions. Ear Hear. *9:* 190–197 (1988).

Fritze, W.: Registration of spontaneous cochlear emissions by means of Fourier transformation. Archs Oto-Rhino-lar. *238:* 189–196 (1983a).

Fritze, W.: On the frequency-distribution of spontaneous cochlear emissions; in Klinke, Hartmann, Hearing – physiological bases and psychophysic, pp. 77–81 (Springer, Berlin 1983b).

Fritze, W.: Spontaneous otoacoustic emissions: their structure and temporal fluctuation. Abstr. Int. Symp. Clinical Applications of Otoacoustic Emissions, Montpellier 1988.

Fritze, W.; Köhler, W.: Frequency composition of spontaneous cochlear emissions. Archs Oto-Rhino-Lar. *242:* 43–48 (1985).

Fritze, W.; Köhler, W.: Our present experience on spontaneous cochlear emissions. Scand. Audiol. *25:* suppl., pp. 129–137.

Furst, M.; Lapid, M.: A cochlear model for acoustic emissions. J. acoust. Soc. Am. *84:* 222–229 (1988).

Furst, M.; Rabinowitz, W.M.; Zurek, P.M.: Ear canal acoustic distortion at $2f_1-f_2$ from human ears: relation to other emissions and perceived combination tones. J. acoust. Soc. Am. *84:* 215–221 (1988).

Gibian, G.L.; Kim, D.O.: Cochlear microphonic evidence for mechanical propagation of distortion products (f_2-f_1) and $(2f_1-f_1)$. Hear. Res. *6:* 35–59 (1982).

Glanville, J.D.; Coles, R.R.A.; Sullivan, B.M.: A family with high-tonal objective tinnitus. J. Lar. Otol. *85:* 1–10 (1971).

Gold, T.: Hearing. II. The physical basis of the action of the cochlea. Proc. R. Soc. Lond. B Biol. Sci. *135:* 492–498 (1948).

Gold, T.; Pumphrey, R.J.: Hearing. I. The cochlea as a frequency analyser. Rroc. R. Soc. Lond. B Biol. Sci. *135:* 462–491 (1948).

Goldstein, J.L.: Auditory nonlinearity. J. acoust. Soc. Am. *41:* 676–689 (1967).

Grandori, F.: Evoked oto-acoustic emissions stimulus-response relationships. Rev. Laryngol. *104:* 153–155 (1983).

Grandori, F.: Nonlinear phenomena in click- and tone-burst-evoked otoacoustic emissions from human ears. Audiology *24:* 71–80 (1985).

Grose, J.H.: The effect of contralateral stimulation on spontaneous acoustic emissions. J. acoust. Soc. Am. *74:* suppl. 1, p. S38 (1983).

Guinan, J.J.: Effect of efferent neural activity on cochlear mechanics. Scand. Audiol. *25:* suppl., pp. 53–61 (1986).

Hall, J.L.: Auditory distortion products f_2-f_1 and $2f_1-f_2$. J. acoust. Soc. Am. *51:* 1863–1871 (1972).

Hammel, D.R.: The frequency of occurrence of spontaneous otoacoustic emissions in normal-hearing young adults; master thesis, Urbana (1983).

Harris, F.P.; Glattke, T.J.: Distortion-product emissions in human with high-frequency sensorineural hearing loss. J. acoust. Soc. Am. *84:* suppl. 1, p. S74 (1988).

Harris, F.P.; Stagner, B.B.; Martin, G.K.; Lonsbury-Martin, B.L.: Effects of frequency separation of primary tones on the amplitude of acoustic distortion products. J. acoust. Soc. Am. *82:* suppl. 1, p. S117 (1987).

Hawkins, J.E.; Johnsson, L.G.: Patterns of sensorineural degeneration in human ears exposed to noise; in Henderson, Hamernik, Dosanjh, Mills, Effects of noise on hearing, pp. 91–100 (Raven Press, New York 1976).

Hawkins, J.E.; Miller, J.M.; Rouse, R.C.; Davis, J.A.; Rarey, K.: Inner ear histopathology in aging rhesus monkeys (*Macaca mulatta*); in Davis, Heathers, Behavior and physiology of aging in rhesus monkeys, pp. 137–154 (Liss, New York 1985).

Hazell, J.W.P.: Spontaneous cochlear acoustic emissions and tinnitus. Clinical experience in the tinnitus patient. J. Lar. Otol. *9:* suppl., pp. 106–110 (1984).

Helmholtz, H.: Die Lehre von den Tonempfindungen, als physiologische Grundlage für die Theorie der Musik. 3. Ausgabe (Vieweg & Sohn, Braunschweig 1870).

Hinz, M.; Wedel, H. von: Otoakustische Emissionen bei Patienten mit Hörsturz. Archs Oto-Rhino-Lar., suppl. II, pp. 128–130 (1984).

Hirsh, I.J.; Bilger, R.C.: Auditory-threshold recovery after exposure to pure tones. J. acoust. Soc. Am. *27:* 1186–1194 (1955).

Horner, K.C.; Lenoir, M.; Bock, G.R.: Distorsion product otoacoustic emissions in hearing-impaired mutant mice. J. acoust. Soc. Am. *78:* 1603–1611 (1985).

Horst, J.W.; Wit, H.P.; Ritsma, R.J.: Psychophysical aspects of cochlear acoustic emissions (Kemp-tones); in Klinke, Hartmann, Hearing – physiological bases and psychophysic, pp. 89–96 (Springer, Berlin 1983).

Hubbard, A.E.; Mountain, D.C.: Alternating current delivered into the scala media alters sound pressure at the eardrum. Science *222:* 510–512 (1983).

Hudspeth, A.J.: The cellular basis of hearing: the biophysics of hair cells. Science *230:* 745–752 (1985a).

Hudspeth, A.J.: Models for mechanoelectrical transduction by hair cells; in Correia, Perachio, Contemporary sensory neurobiology, pp. 193–205 (Liss, New York 1985b).

Huizing, E.H.; Spoor, A.: An unusual type of tinnitus. Archs Otolar. *98:* 134–136 (1973).

Humes, L.E.: Psychophysical measures of two-tone suppression and distortion products $(2f_1-f_2)$ and (f_2-f_1). J. acoust. Soc. Am. *73:* 930–950 (1983).

Humes, L.E.: An excitation-pattern algorithm for the estimation of $(2f_1-f_2)$ and (f_2-f_1) cancellation level and phase. J. acoust. Soc. Am. *78:* 1252–1260 (1985).

Johnsen, N.J.; Bagi, P.; Elberling, C.: Evoked acoustic emissions from the human ear. III. Findings in neonates. Scand. Audiol. *12:* 17–24 (1983).

Johnsen, N.J.; Bagi, P.; Parbo, J.; Elberling, C.: Evoked acoustic emissions from the human ear. IV. Final result in 100 neonates. Scand. Audiol. *17:* 27–34 (1988).

Johnsen, N.J.; Elberling, C.: Evoked acoustic emissions from the human ear. I. Equipment and response parameters. Scand. Audiol. *11:* 3–12 (1982a).

Johnsen, N.J.; Elberling, C.: Evoked acoustic emissions from the human ear. II. Normative data in young adults and influence of posture. Scand. Audiol. *11:* 69–77 (1982b).

Jones, K.; Tubis, A.; Long, G.R.; Burns, E.M.; Strickland, E.A.: Interactions among multiple spontaneous otoacoustic emissions; in Allen, Hall, Hubbard, Neely, Tubis, Peripheral auditory mechanisms, pp. 266–273 (Springer, Berlin 1986).

Kemp, D.T.: Stimulated acoustic emissions from within the human auditory system. J. acoust. Soc. Am. *64:* 1386–1391 (1978).

Kemp, D.T.: Evidence of mechanical nonlinearity and frequency selective wave amplification in the cochlea. Archs Oto-Rhino-Lar. *224:* 37–45 (1979a).

Kemp, D.T.: The evoked cochlear mechanical responses and the auditory microstructure – evidence for a new element in cochlear mechanics. Scand. Audiol. *9:* suppl., pp. 35–47 (1979b).

Kemp, D.T.: Towards a model for the origin of cochlear echoes. Hear. Res. *2:* 533–548 (1980).

Kemp, D.T.: Physiologically active cochlear micromechanics – one source of tinnitus; in Evered, Lawrenson, Tinnitus. Ciba Fdn Symp., pp. 54–81 (Pitman, London 1981).

Kemp, D.T.: Cochlear echoes: implications for noise-induced hearing loss; in Hamernik, Henderson, Salvi, New perspectives on noise-induced hearing loss, pp. 189–207 (Raven Press, New York 1982).

Kemp, D.T.: Otoacoustic emissions, traveling waves and cochlear mechanisms. Hear. Res. *22:* 95–104 (1986).

Kemp, D.T.: Developments in cochlear mechanics and techniques for noninvasive evaluation. Adv. Audiol. *5:* 27–45 (1988).

Kemp, D.T.; Bray, P.; Alexander, L.; Brown, A.M.: Acoustic emission cochleography – practical aspects. Scand. Audiol. *25:* suppl., pp. 71–82 (1986).

Kemp, D.T.; Brown, A.M.: A comparison of mechanical nonlinearities in the cochleae of man and gerbil from ear canal measurements; in Klinke, Hartmann, Hearing – physiological bases and psychophysic, pp. 82–88 (Springer, Berlin 1983a).

Kemp, D.T.; Brown, A.M.: An integrated view of cochlear mechanical nonlinearities observable from the ear canal; in de Boer, Viergever, Mechanics of hearing, pp. 75–82 (Nijhoff, The Hague 1983b).

Kemp, D.T.; Brown, A.M.: Ear canal acoustic and round window electrical correlates of $2f_1-f_2$ distortion generated in the cochlea. Hear. Res. *13:* 39–46 (1984).

Kemp, D.T.; Brown, A.M.: Wideband analysis of otoacoustic intermodulation; in Allen, Hall, Hubbard, Neely, Tubis, Peripheral auditory mechanisms, pp. 306–313 (Springer, Berlin 1986).

Kemp, D.T.; Chum, R.A.: Observations on the generator mechanism of stimulus frequency acoustic emissions – two-tone suppression; in van den Brink, Bilsen, Psychophysical, physiological, and behavioral studies in hearing, pp. 34–42 (Delft University Press, Delft 1980a).

Kemp, D.T.; Chum, R.A.: Properties of the generator of stimulated acoustic emissions. Hear. Res. *2:* 213–232 (1980b).

Kemp, D.T.; Souter, M.: A new rapid component in the cochlear response to brief electrical efferent stimulation: CM and otoacoustic observations. Hear. Res. *34:* 49–62 (1988).

Khanna, S.M.; Leonard, D.G.B.: Basilar membrane tuning in the cat cochlea. Science *215:* 305–306 (1982).

Kim, D.O.: A review of nonlinear and active cochlear models; in Allen, Hall, Hubbard, Neely, Tubis, Peripheral auditory mechanisms, pp. 239–247 (Springer, Berlin 1986a).

Kim, D.O.: Active and nonlinear cochlear biomechanics and the role of outer-hair-cell subsystem in the mammalian auditory system. Hear. Res. *22:* 105–114 (1986b).

Kim, D.O.; Molnar, C.E.; Matthews, J.W.: Cochlear mechanics: nonlinear behavior in two-tone responses as reflected in cochlear-nerve-fiber responses and in ear-canal sound pressure. J. acoust. Soc. Am. *67:* 1704–1721 (1980).

Klinke, R.: Die Verarbeitung von Schallreizen im Innenohr – Eine Übersicht über neuere Forschungsergebnisse. HNO *35:* 139–148 (1987).

Köhler, W.; Fredriksen, E.; Fritze, W.: Spontaneous otoacoustic emissions – a comparison of the left versus right ear. Archs Oto-Rhino-Lar. *243:* 43–46 (1986).

Kössl, M.; Vater, M.: Evoked acoustic emissions and cochlear microphonics in the mustache bat, *Pteronotus parnellii*. Hear. Res. *19:* 157–170 (1985).

Kumpf, W.; Hoke, M.: Ein konstantes Ohrgeräusch bei 4000 Hz. Arch. klin. exp. Ohr.-Nas.-KehlkHeilk. *196:* 243–247 (1970).

Lenoir, M.; Puel, J.-L.: Development of $2f_1 - f_2$ otoacoustic emissions in the rat. Hear. Res. *29:* 265–271 (1987).

Lewis, E.R.: Speculations about noise and the evolution of vertebrate hearing. Hear. Res. *25:* 83–90 (1987).

Lim, D.J.: Functional structure of the organ of Corti: a review. Hear. Res. *22:* 117–146 (1986).

Lippe, R.W.: Recent developments in cochlear physiology. Ear Hear. *7:* 233–239 (1986).

Loebell, E.: Krankendemonstrationen. HNO *10:* 222 (1962).

Long, G.R.; Tubis, A.: Modification of spontaneous and evoked otoacoustic emissions and associated psychoacoustic microstructure by aspirin consumption. J. acoust. Soc. Am. *84:* 1343–1353 (1988).

Long, G.R.; Tubis, A.; Jones, K.: Changes in spontaneous and evoked otoacoustic emissions and corresponding psychoacoustic threshold microstructures induced by aspirin consumption; in Allen, Hall, Hubbard, Neely, Tubis, Peripheral auditory mechanisms, pp. 213–220 (Springer, Berlin 1986).

Lonsbury-Martin, B.L.; Harris, F.P.; Hawkins, M.D.; Stagner, B.B.; Martin, G.K.: Acoustic distortion products in humans. Abstr. 11th Midwinter Research Meet. Ass. Res. Otolaryngol., 1988a, p. 178.

Lonsbury-Martin, B.L.; Martin, G.K.: Incidence of spontaneous otoacoustic emissions in macaque monkeys: a replication. Hear. Res. *34:* 313–317 (1988).

Lonsbury-Martin, B.L.; Martin, G.K.; Probst, R.; Coats, A.C.: Acoustic distorsion products in rabbit ear canal. I. Basic features and physilogical vulnerability. Hear. Res. *28:* 173–189 (1987).

Lonsbury-Martin, B.L.; Martin, G.K.; Probst, R.; Coats, A.C.: Spontaneous otoacoustic emissions in a nonhuman primate. II. Cochlear anatomy. Hear. Res. *33:* 69–94 (1988b).

Lumer, G.: Computer model for cochlear preprocessing (steady state condition). I. Basics and results for one sinusoidal input signal. Acustica *62:* 282–290 (1987a).

Lumer, G.: Computer model for cochlear preprocessing (steady-state condition). II. Two-tone suppression. Acustica *63:* 17–25 (1987b).

Lutman, M.E.; Fleming, A.J.: Sensitivity and specificity of click evoked otoacoustic emissions as screening test for normal cochlear function. Abstr. Int. Symp. Clinical Applications of Otoacoustic Emissions, Montpellier 1988.

Manley, G.A.: Frequency spacing of acoustic emissions: a possible explanation; in Webster, Mechanisms of hearing, pp. 36–39 (Monash University Press, Clayton, 1983).

Manley, G.A.; Schulze, M.; Oeckinghaus, H.: Otoacoustic emissions in a song bird. Hear. Res. *26:* 257–266 (1987).

Martin, G.K.; Lonsbury-Martin, B.L.; Probst, R.; Coats, A.C.: Spontaneous otoacoustic emissions in the nonhuman primate: a survey. Hear. Res. *20:* 91–95 (1985).

Martin, G.K.; Lonsbury-Martin, B.L.; Probst, R.; Coats, A.C.: Acoustic distorsion products in rabbit ear canal. II. Sites of origin revealed by suppression contours and pure-tone exposures. Hear. Res. *28:* 191–108 (1987a).

Martin, G.K.; Lonsbury-Martin, B.L.; Stagner, B.B.; Coats, A.C.: Alteration in behavior thresholds, acoustic distortion products, and summating potentials following experimentally induced endolymphatic hydrops in rabbit. Abstr. 10th Midwinter Research Meet. Ass. Res. Otolaryngol., 1987b, p. 18.

Martin, G.K.; Lonsbury-Martin, B.L.; Probst, R.; Coats, A.C.: Spontaneous otoacoustic emissions in a nonhuman primate. I. Basic features and relations to other emissions. Hear. Res. *33:* 49–68 (1988).

Matthews, J.W.: Modeling reverse middle ear transmission of acoustic distorsion signals; in de Boer, Viergever, Mechanics of hearing, pp. 11–18 (Nijhoff, The Hague 1983).

Matthews, J.W.; Molnar, C.E.: Modeling intracochlear and ear canal distortion product $(2f_1-f_2)$; in Allen, Hall, Hubbard, Neely, Tubis, Peripheral auditory mechanisms, pp. 258–265 (Springer, Berlin 1986).

McFadden, D.; Plattsmier, H.S.: Aspirin abolishes spontaneous oto-acoustic emissions. J. acoust. Soc. Am. *76:* 443–448 (1984).

McFadden, D.; Plattsmier, H.S.; Pasanen, E.G.: Aspirin-induced hearing loss as a model of sensorineural hearing loss. Hear. Res. *16:* 251–260 (1984).

McFadden, D.; Wightman, F.L.: Audition: some relations between normal and pathological hearing. A. Rev. Psychol. *34:* 95–128 (1983).

Mott, J.B.; Norton, S.J.; Neely, S.T.; Warr, W.B.: Changes in spontaneous otoacoustic emissions produced by acoustic stimulation of the contralateral ear. Abst. 10th Midwinter Research Meet. Ass. Res. Otolaryngol, 1987, p. 21.

Mountain, D.C.: Changes in endolymphatic potential and crossed olivocochlear bundle stimulation alters cochlear mechanics. Science *210:* 71–72 (1980).

Mountain, D.C.: Active filtering by hair cells; in Allen, Hall, Hubbard, Neely, Tubis, Peripheral auditory mechanisms, pp. 179–188 (Springer, Berlin 1986).

Mountain, D.C.; Hubbard, A.E.; McMullen, T.A.: Electromechanical processes in the cochlea; in Klinke, Hartmann, Hearing – physiological bases and psychophysic, pp. 119–126 (Springer, Berlin 1983).

Neely, S.T.; Kim, D.O.: A model for active elements in cochlear biomechanics. J. acoust. Soc. Am. *79:* 1472–1480 (1986).

Neely, S.T.; Norton, S.J.; Gorga, M.P.; Jestead, W.: Latency of otoacoustic emissions and ABR wave V using tone-burst stimuli. J. acoust. Soc. Am. *79:* suppl. 1, p. S5 (1986).

Neely, S.T.; Norton, S.J.; Gorga, M.P.; Jestead, W.: Latency of auditory brain-stem responses and otoacoustic emissions using tone-burst stimuli. J. acoust. Soc. Am. *83:* 652–656 (1988).

Norton, S.J.; Champlin, C.A.; Mott, J.B.: Effect of intense sound exposure on spontaneous otoacoustic emissions. J. acoust. Soc. Am. *79:* suppl. 1, p. S5 (1986).

Norton, S.J.; Champlin, C.A.; Mott, J.B.: The behavior of spontaneous otoacoustic emissions from human ears following exposure to intense pure-tone stimuli. Abstr. 10th Midwinter Research Meet. Ass. Res. Otolaryngol., 1987, p. 21.

Norton, S.J.; Mott, J.B.: Effects of auditory fatigue on psychophysical estimates of cochlear nonlinearities. J. acoust. Soc. Am. *82:* 80–87 (1987).

Norton, S.J.; Neely, S.T.: Latency of click-evoked otoacoustic emissions in humans. Abstr. 8th Midwinter Research Meet. Ass. Res. Otolaryngol, 1985, p. 79.

Norton, D.J.; Neely, S.T.: Tone-burst-evoked otoacoustic emissions from normal-hearing subjects. J. acoust. Soc. Am. *81:* 1860–1872 (1987).

Palmer, A.R.; Wilson, J.P.: Spontaneous and evoked acoustic emissions in the frog *Rana esculenta.* J. Physiol. *324:* 66 (1982).

Penner, M.J.; Burns, E.M.: The dissociation of SOAEs and tinnitus. J. Speech Hear. Res. *30:* 396–403 (1987).

Pickles, J.O.: Recent advances in cochlear physiology. Prog. Neurobio. *24:* 1–42 (1985).

Plomp, R.: Detectability thresholds for combination tones. J. acoust. Soc. Am. *37:* 1110–1123 (1965).

Probst, R.; Antonelli, C.; Pieren, C.: Methods and preliminary results of distortion product otoacoustic emissions in normal and pathological ears. Abstr. 2nd Int. Conf. Cochlear Mechanics and Otoacoustic Emissions, Rome 1989.

Probst, R.; Beck, D.: Influence of general anesthesia on spontaneous otoacoustic emissions. Abstr. 10th Midwinter Research Meet. Ass. Res. Otolaryngol., 1987, p. 17.

Probst, R.; Coats, A.C.; Martin, G.K.; Lonsbury-Martin, B.L.: Spontaneous, click-, and toneburst-evoked otoacoustic emissions from normal ears. Hear. Res. *21:* 261–275 (1986).

Probst, R.; Lonsbury-Martin, B.L.; Martin, G.K.; Coats, A.C.: Otoacoustic emissions in ears with hearing loss. Am. J. Otolaryngol. *8:* 73–81 (1987).

Rabinowitz, W.M.; Widin, G.P.: Interaction of spontaneous oto-acoustic emissions and external sounds. J. acoust. Soc. Am. *76:* 1713–1720 (1984).

Rebilliard, G.; Abbou, S.; Lenoir, M.: Les oto-émissions acoustiques. II. Les oto-émissions spontanées: résultats chez des sujets normaux ou présentant des acouphènes. Annls Oto-lar. *104:* 363–368 (1987).

Rosowski, J.J.; Peake, W.T.; Lynch, T.J.: Acoustic input-admittance of the alligator-lizare ear: nonlinear features. Hear. Res. *16:* 205–223 (1984a).

Rosowski, J.J.; Peake, W.T.; White, J.R.: Cochlear nonlinearities inferred from two-tone distorsion products in the ear canal of the alligator lizard. Hear. Res. *13:* 141–158 (1984b).

Ruggero, M.A.; Kramek, B.; Rich, N.C.: Spontaneous otoacoustic emissions in a dog. Hear. Res. *13:* 293–296 (1984).

Ruggero, M.A.; Rich, N.C.; Freyman, R.: Spontaneous and impulsively evoked otoacoustic emissions: Indicators of cochlear pathology? Hear. Res. *10:* 283–300 (1983).

Rutten, W.L.C.: Evoked acoustic emissions from within normal and abnormal human ears: comparison with audiometric and electrocochleographic findings. Hear. Res. *2:* 263–271 (1980a).

Rutten, W.L.C.: Latencies of stimulated acoustic emissions in normal human ears, in van den Brink, Bilsen, Psychophysical, physiological, and behavioral studies in hearing, pp. 68–76 (Delft University Press, Delft 1980b).

Rutten, W.L.C.; Buisman, H.P.: Critical behaviour of auditory oscillators near feedback phase transitions; in de Boer, Viergever, Mechanics of hearing, pp. 91–99 (Nijhoff, The Hague 1983).

Scherer, A.: Evozierte oto-akustische Emissionen bei Vor- und Nachverdeckung. Acustica *56:* 34–40 (1984).

Schloth, E.: Akustische Aussendungen des menschilchen Ohres (oto-akustische Emissionen); Dissertation, München (1982).

Schloth, E.: Relation between spectral composition of spontaneous otoacoustic emissions and fine-structure of threshold in quiet. Acustica *53:* 250–256 (1983).

Schloth, E; Zwicker, E.: Mechanical and acoustical influences on spontaneous oto-acoustic emission. Hear. Res. *11:* 285–293 (1983).

Schmiedt, R.A.: Acoustic distorsion in the ear canal. I. Cubic difference tones: effects of acute noise injury. J. acoust. Soc. Am. *79:* 1481–1490 (1986a).

Schmiedt, R.A.: Harmonic acoustic emissions in the earcanal generated by single tones: experiments and a model; in Allen, Hall, Hubbard, Neely, Tubis, Peripheral auditory mechanisms, pp. 330–337 (Springer, Berlin 1986b).

Schmiedt, R.A.: Effects of asphyxia on levels of ear canal emissions in gerbils. Abstr. 9th Midwinter Research Meet. Ass. Res. Otolaryngol., 1986c, p. 112.

Schmiedt, R.A.; Adams, J.C.: Stimulated acoustic emissions in the ear of the gerbil. Hear. Res. *5:* 295–305 (1981).

Schmiedt, R.A.; Addy, C.L.: Ear-canal acoustic emissions as frequency specific indicators of cochlear function. J. acoust. Soc. Am. *72:* suppl. 1, p. S6 (1982).

Sellick, P.M.; Patuzzi, R.; Johnstone, B.M.: Measurement of basilar membrane motion in the guinea pig using the Mössbauer technique. J. acoust. Soc. Am. *72:* 131–141 (1982).

Siegel, J.H.; Kim, D.O.: Cochlear biomechanics: vulnerability to acoustic trauma and other alterations as seen in neural responses and ear-canal sound pressure, in Hamernik, Henderson, Salvi, New perspectives on noise-induced hearing loss, pp. 137–151 (Raven Press, New York 1982a).

Siegel, J.H.; Kim, D.O.: Efferent neural control of cochlear mechanics? Olivocochlear bundle stimulation affects cochlear biomechanical nonlinearity. Hear. Res. *6:* 171–182 (1982b).

Siegel, J.H.; Kim, D.O.; Molnar, C.E.: Effects of altering organ of Corti on cochlear distortion products f_2-f_1 and $2f_1-f_2$. J. Neurophysiol. *47:* 303–328 (1982).

Smoorenburg, G.F.: Combination tones and their origin. J. acoust. Soc. Am. *52:* 615–632 (1972).

Stainback, R.F.; Lonsbury-Martin, B.L.; Martin, G.K.; Coats, A.C.: Noise damage and its relation to acoustic distrotion-product generation in the rabbit. Abstr. 10th Midwinter Research Meet. Ass. Res. Otolaryngol., 1987, p. 19.

Stevens, J.C.: Click-evoked oto-acoustic emissions in normal and hearing-impaired adults. Br. J. Audiol. *22:* 42–49 (1988).

Stevens, J.C.; Webb, H.D.; Hutchinson, J.; Connell, J.; Smith, M.F.; Buffin, J.T.: A prospective study of the application of click evoked otoacoustic emissions to detect hearing impairment at birth. Abstr. Int. Symp. Clinical Applications of Otoacoustic Emissions, Montpellier 1988.

Stevens, J.C.; Webb, H.D.; Smith, M.F.; Buffin, J.T.; Ruddy, H.: A comparison of oto-acoustic emissions and brain stem electric response audiometry in the normal newborn and babies admitted to a special care baby unit. Clin. Phys. Physiol. Meas. *8:* 95–104 (1987).

Strack, G.: Untersuchungen auf oto-akustische Emissionen aus dem Innenohr des Brillenkaimans (*Caiman crocodilus*); Dissertation, Frankfurt (1986).

Strickland, A.E.; Burns, E.M.; Tubis, A.; Jones, K.: Long-term stability and familial aspects of spontaneous otoacoustic emissions. J. acoust. Soc. Am. *75:* suppl. 1, p. S82 (1984).

Strickland, A.E.; Burns, E.M.; Tubis, A.: Incidence of spontaneous otoacoustic emissions in children and infants. J. acoust. Soc. Am. *78:* 931–935 (1985).

Sutton, G.J.; Wilson, J.P.: Modelling cochlear echoes: the influence of irregularities in frequency mapping on summed cochlear activity; in de Boer, Viergever, Mechanics of hearing, pp. 83–90 (Nijhoff, The Hague 1983).

Tinnitus: Appendix I. Definition and classification of tinnitus, pp. 300–302 (Pitman, London 1981).

Thornton, A.R.D.: Evoked otoacoustic emissions in neonates. Abstr. Int. Symp. Clinical Applications of Otoacoustic Emissions, Montpellier 1988.

Tyler, R.S.; Conrad-Armes, D.: Spontaneous acoustic cochlear emissions and sensorineural tinnitus. Br. J. Audiol. *16:* 193–194 (1982).

Uziel, A.; Bonfils, P.: Otoacoustic emissions in sensorineural hearing loss and retrocochlear disease. Abstr. Int. Symp. Clinical Applications of Otoacoustic Emissions, Montpellier 1988.

Weber, R.; Mellert, V.: On the non-monotonic behaviour of cubic distortion products in the human ear. J. acoust. Soc. Am. *57:* 207–214 (1975).

Weiss, T.F.: Bidirectional transduction in vertebrate hair cells: a mechanism for coupling mechanical and electrical processes. Hear. Res. *7:* 353–360 (1982).

Wenner, C.H.: Intensities of aural difference tones. J. acoust. Soc. Am. *43:* 77–80 (1968).

Wever, E.G.; Bray, C.W.; Lawrence, M.: The interference of tones in the cochlea. J. acoust. Soc. Am. *12:* 268–280 (1940).

Wiederhold, M.L.; Mahoney, J.W.; Kellogg, D.L.: Acoustic overstimulation reduces $2f_1-f_2$ cochlear emissions at all levels in the cat; in Allen, Hall, Hubbard, Neely, Tubis, Peripheral auditory mechanisms, pp. 322–329 (Springer, Berlin 1986).

Wier, C.C.; Norton, S.J.; Kincaid, G.E.: Spontaneous narrow-band oto-acoustic signals emitted by human ears: a replication. J. acoust. Soc. Am. *76:* 1248–1250 (1984).

Wier, C.C.; Pasanen, E.G.; McFadden, D.: Partial dissociation of spontaneous otoacoustic emissions and distortion products during aspirin use in humans. J. acoust. Soc. Am. *84:* 230–237 (1988).

Wilson, J.P.: Evidence for a cochlear origin for acoustic re-emissions, threshold fine-structure and tonal tinnitus. Hear. Res. *2:* 233–252 (1980a).

Wilson, J.P.: Subthreshold mechanical activity within the cochlea. J. Physiol *298:* P 32–33 (1980b).

Wilson, J.P.: Model for cochlear echoes and tinnitus based on an observed electrical correlate. Hear. Res. *2:* 527–532 (1980c).

Wilson, J.P.: The combination tone, $2f_1-f_2$, in psychophysics and ear-canal recording; in van den Brink, Bilsen, Psychophysical, physiological, and behavioral studies in hearing, pp. 43–52 (Delft University Press, Delft 1980d).

Wilson, J.P.: Otoacoustic emissions and hearing mechanisms. Rev. Laryngol. *105:* 179–191 (1984).

Wilson, J.P.; The influence of temperature on frequency-tuning mechanisms; in Allen, Hall, Hubbard, Neely, Tubis, Peripheral auditory mechanisms, pp. 229–236 (Springer, Berlin 1986a).

Wilson, J.P.: Otoacoustic emissions and tinnitus. Scand. Audiol. *25:* suppl., pp. 109–119 (1986b).

Wilson, J.P.; Evans, E.F.: Effects of furosemide, flaxedil, noise and tone over-stimulation on the evoked otoacoustic emission in cat. Proc. Int. Union Physiol. Sc. *XV:* 100 (1983).

Wilson, J.P.; Sutton, G.J.: acoustic correlates of tonal tinnitus; in Evered, Lawrenson, Tinnitus. Ciba Fdn. Symp., pp. 82–107 (Pitman, London 1981).

Wilson, J.P.; Sutton, G.J.: A family with high-tonal objective tinnitus–an update; in Klinke, Hartmann, Hearing – physiological bases and psychophysic, pp. 97–103 (Springer, Berlin 1983).

Wit, H.P.: Diurnal cycle for spontaneous oto-acoustic emission frequency. Hear. Res. *18:* 197–199 (1985).

Wit, H.P.: Statistical properties of a strong spontaneous oto-acoustic emission; in Allen, Hall, Hubbard, Neely, Tubis, Peripheral auditory mechanisms, pp. 221–228 (Springer, Berlin 1986).

Wit, H.P.; Kahmann, H.F.: Frequency analysis of stimulated cochlear acoustic emissions in monkey ears. Hear. Res. *8:* 1–11 (1982).

Wit, H.P.; Langevoort, J.C.; Ritsma, R.J.: Frequency spectra of cochlear acoustic emissions (Kemp-echoes). J. acoust. Soc. Am. *70:* 437–445 (1981).

Wit, H.P.; Ritsma, R.J.: Stimulated acoustic emissions from the human ear. J. acoust. Soc. Am. *66:* 911–913 (1979).

Wit, H.P.; Ritsma, R.J.: Evoked acoustical responses from the human ear: some experimental results. Hear. Res. *2:* 253–261 (1980).

Wit, H.P.; Ritsma, R.J.: Two aspects of cochlear acoustic emissions: response latency and minimum stimulus energy; in de Boer, Viergever, Mechanics of hearing, pp. 101–107 (Nijhoff, The Hague 1983a).

Wit, H.P.; Ritsma, R.J.: Sound emission from the ear triggered by single molecules? Neurosci. Lett. *40:* 275–280 (1983b).

Yamamoto, E.; Takagi, A.; Hirono, Y.; Yagi, N.: A case of 'spontaneous otoacoustic emission'. Archs Otolaryngol. Head Neck Surg. *113:* 1316–1318 (1987).

Yates, G.K.; Bishop, P.: Cochlear echoes in guinea pigs. Ann. Report 3, p. 14 (Institute of Hearing Research, Nottingham 1979).

Zenner, H.P.; Gitter, A.H.: Die Schallverarbeitung des Ohres. Physik unserer Zeit *18:* 97–105

Zenner, H.P.; Zimmermann, U.; Gitter, A.H.: Fast motility of isolated mammalian auditory sensory cells. Biochem. biophys. Res. Commun. *149:* (1987).

Zurek, P.M.: Spontaneous narrowband acoustic signals emitted by human ears. J. acoust. Soc. Am. *69:* 514–523 (1981).

Zurek, P.M.; Clark, W.W.: Narrow-band acoustic signals emitted by chinchilla ears after noise exposure. J. acoust. Soc. Am. *70:* 446–450 (1981).

Zurek, P.M.; Clark, W.W.; Kim, D.O.: The behavior of acoustic distorsion products in the ear canals of chinchillas with normal or damaged ears. J. acoust. Soc. Am. *72:* 774–780 (1982).

Zurek, P.M.; Leshowitz, B.H.: Measurement of the combination tone f_2-f_1 and $2f_1-f_2$. J. acoust. Soc. Am. *61:* 155–168 (1976).

Zwicker, E.: Der ungewöhnliche Amplitudengang der nichtlinearen Verzerrung des Ohres. Acustica *5:* 67–74 (1955).

Zwicker, E.: A model describing nonlinearities in hearing by active processes with saturation at 40 dB. Biol. Cybernet. *35:* 243–250 (1979a).

Zwicker, E.: Different behavior of quadratic and cubic difference tones. Hear. Res. *1:* 283–292 (1979b).

Zwicker, E.: Nonmonotonic behavior of $(2f_1-f_2)$ explained by a saturation-feedback model. Hear. Res. *2:* 513–518 (1980a).

Zwicker, E.: Cubic difference tone level and phase dependence on frequency difference and level of primaries; in van den Brink, Bilsen, Psychophysical, physiological, and behavioral studies in hearing, pp. 268–271 (Delft University Press, Delft 1980b).

Zwicker, E.: Masking-period patterns and cochlear acoustical responses. Hear. Res. *4:* 195–202 (1981a).

Zwicker, E.: Dependence of level and phase of the $(2f_1-f_2)$-cancellation tone on frequency range, frequency difference, level of primaries, and subject. J. acoust. Soc. Am. *70:* 1277–1288 (1981b).

Zwicker, E.: Delayed evoked oto-acoustic emissions and their suppression by Gaussian-shaped pressure impulses. Hear. Res. *11:* 359–371 (1983a).

Zwicker, E.: On peripheral processing in human hearing; in Klinke, Hartmann, Hearing – physiological bases and psychophysic, pp. 104–110 (Springer, Berlin 1983b).

Zwicker, E.: A hardware cochlear nonlinear preprocessing model with active feedback. J. acoust. Soc. Am. *80:* 146–153 (1986a).

Zwicker, E.: Otoacoustic emissions in a nonlinear cochlear hardware model with feedback. J. acoust. Soc. Am. *80:* 154–162 (1986b).

Zwicker, E.: Suppression and $(2f_1-f_2)$-difference tones in a nonlinear cochlear preprocessing model with active feedback. J. acoust. Soc. Am. *80:* (1986c).

Zwicker, E.; Manley, G.: Acoustical responses and suppression-period patterns in guinea pigs. Hear. Res. *4:* 43–52 (1981).

Zwicker, E.; Schloth, E.: Interrelation of different oto-acoustic emissions. J. acoust. Soc. Am. *75:* 1148–1154 (1984).

Zwicker, E.; Stecker, M.; Hind, J.: Relations between masking, otoacoustic emissions, and evoked potential. Acustica *64:* 102–109 (1987).

Zwislocki, J.: Analysis of middle ear function. I. Input impedance. J. acoust. Soc. Am. *34:*1514–1523 (1962).

Zwislocki, J.J.: How OHC lesions can lead to neural cochlear hypersensitivity. Acta oto-lar. *97:* 529–534 (1984).

Zwislocki, J.J.: Cochlear function–an analysis. Acta oto-lar. *100:* 201–209 (1985).

R. Probst, MD, Department of Otorhinolaryngology, Kantonsspital,
University of Basel, CH-4031 Basel (Switzerland)

Pfaltz CR (ed): New Aspects of Cochlear Mechanics and Inner Ear Pathophysiology.
Adv Otorhinolaryngol. Basel, Karger, 1990, vol 44, pp 92–164

Ototoxicity of Loop Diuretics

Morphological and Electrophysiological Examinations in
Animal Experiments[1]

Christian Peter Hommerich

ENT-Clinic (Director: Prof. Dr. K.-H. Vosteen), University of Düsseldorf,
Düsseldorf, FRG

1. Introduction

Damage to the inner ear was first observed as a secondary effect by the
application of streptomycin and dehydrostreptomycin [Brown and Hinshu,
1946; Molitor et al., 1946]. In the following years, this specific organ-
toxicity was also noticed in other aminoglycosides and the term ototoxicity
was subsequently developed for these drugs. One already had differentiated
between two different effects: one on the vestibular organ (streptomycin) and
one on the acoustic organ (dehydrostreptomycin) [Causse, 1949; Farrington
et al., 1947; Ruedi et al., 1952; Shambaugh et al., 1959; Spöndlin, 1966].

A loss of the outer and inner hair cells and of the sensory cells of the
vestibular organ in humans as well as in animal experiments was found as
a morphological correlate of these hearing and vestibular disturbances
[Duvall and Wersäll, 1964; Spöndlin, 1966; Duvall and Quick, 1969; Wersäll
et al., 1973]. In accordance with the decreasing threshold curve in the human
audiogram, a functional loss with the decrease of the cochlea microphonics
and the compound action potentials (CAP) after streptomycin administration could also be observed in animal experiments. However, the ductus
cochlearis (DC) potential of the endolymph did not change. The sensory
neural hearing impairment after aminoglycoside application was usually
pancochlear, dose-dependent and always irreversible.

After the introduction of loop diuretics such as ethacrynic acid (EA)
and other drugs with a similar mechanism, hearing impairment of patients
was also observed. Maher and Schreiner [1965] first described this phenomenon which was later to be confirmed by other publications [Schneider

---

[1]Dedicated to my father.

and Becker, 1966; Vargish et al., 1970; Mathog et al., 1970; Schwarz et al., 1970; Matz, 1976]. These observations were seen in patients with reduced renal function, uremia, or after extremely high doses of loop diuretics.

On the other hand, there are very few publications on clinical observations of functional disturbances of the vestibular organ after administration of diuretics [Schneider and Becker, 1966; Schwarz et al., 1970; Gomolin and Garshik, 1980]. Having observed that the human hearing threshold decreased after diuretics administration under these specific conditions, it was concluded that this drug category was also ototoxic. Unlike the aminoglycoside antibiotics, however, it is to be noted that the ototoxicity upon sole administration of these substances is minimal. As a rule, the hearing impairments are almost always reversible. Audiometrically, the losses can usually be detected at 2–4 kHz [Lehnhardt, 1984]. Functionally, an acute change of the CAP was described [Kuijpers and Bonting, 1970; Brown and McElwee, 1972; Brown, 1975; Aran and de Sauvage, 1977; Syka and Melichar, 1981].

Regarding the target of attack of the loop diuretics in the inner ear, the hair cells initially became the subject of animal experiments [Haubrich and Schätzle, 1970, 1971; Kohonen et al., 1970]. Following EA administration, damage appeared in the outer, but not in the inner hair cells. With more precise investigation of other epithelia of the inner ear, it was proven that this destruction of hair cells was simply a secondary effect of the diuretics. Quick and Duvall [1970] were the first to prove that the stria vascularis was the main site of attack of the EA. In their classical electronmicroscope study of guinea pigs, they presented impressive results which documented a pronounced interstitial edema between the intermediate cells of the stria vascularis with a concomitant hydrops of the marginal cells after application of EA.

These characteristics changes were also described later by other authors [Nakai, 1971; Bosher et al., 1973; Bosher, 1979, 1980]. In animal experiments imitating clinical conditions, a rapid decline of the DC potential from $+80$ to -40 mV, a decrease of the potassium concentration and an increase of the sodium concentration as well as a slight decline of the chloride concentration could be observed in the endolymph. These changes were reversible [Bosher et al., 1973; Bosher, 1979].

Apparently the above electrolyte imbalances are in compliance with the morphological findings in the stria vasularis as the result of EA, because under the electron microscope the cell architecture as well as the cellular organelles of the stria vascularis imply their functional involvement in the electrolyte and water transport; the morphological alterations of the stria correlated with the functional impairment.

Similar morphological conditions are to be found in the secretory epithelia of the ampulla. For this reason, they have been compared repeatedly in the literature with the stria vascularis [Dohlmann, 1964; Kimura et al., 1964; Kimura, 1969; Hiraide, 1971]. Here, a correlation between morphology and function may also exist. In animal experiments, Mathog [1977] demonstrated that apparently a temporary impairment of the vestibular function occurs after EA administration. In his experiments there was a decline of the nystagmus induced by caloric stimulation. Similar effects have also been reported by other authors [Levinson et al., 1974; Kusakari et al., 1979].

Despite these evident findings, the functional alterations of the semi-circular canal and the ampulla of guinea pigs after administration of EA seemed to differ from the cochlear changes. Up to 40 min after injection, in experiments by Sellick and Johnstone [1974], there were no changes in the utriculus potential. Recently, Mori and Morgenstern [1985] additionally found that in the semicircular canal of the guinea pig, the decline of the DC potential after the administration of EA is only very slight and first occurs after 40–50 min.

These contradictory results of the quoted authors motivated us to examine the possibility of morphological alterations in the ampulla and the semicircular canal as a result of the administration of loop diuretics, and to determine whether or not these alterations correlate with physiological changes. In addition, a comparison of the cochlear with the vestibular effect of the loop diuretics seemed a good method for settling the question of whether the term ototoxicity, which pertains to the complete inner ear, can also be applied to loop diuretics in the currently valid universal form. By comparing morphological and electrophysiological investigations of the cochlea and the vestibular organ, it became possible to define and differentiate the toxic effect of EA on the cochlea with that of the vestibular organ. These examinations were carried out on guinea pigs.

The investigations presented were initiated with a reliability and validity test of the applied method by investigating the effect of EA on the cochlea of the guinea pig. Such tests already carried out by other authors in similar experiments allow a comparison of the findings with corresponding literature sources and thereby a statement as to the reproducibility of an 'ethacrynic acid intoxication'.

According to the literature, it was assumed that loop diuretics only slightly affected the secretory epithelia of the ampulla of guinea pigs. In order also to obtain more precise information about the effect of the EA on this labyrinthine component, we deviated from the conventional experimental setup in this area and changed the animal species, using pigeons to investigate the influence of the EA on the ampulla. The pigeon is ideal for such experiments because it has a well-developed vestibular organ [Dohlmann, 1970, 1980].

In addition, we expected to gain information by comparing investigations on the cochlea of the pigeon with those on guinea pigs in regard to the different effects of the loop diuretics on the cochlear components of each animal. According to results obtained until now, it may be assumed that, for the guinea pig, the stria vascularis is predominantly sensitive to the loop diuretics and that the vestibular apparatus is only minimally affected. With the animal experiment, support for this hypothesis could be gained, if in appropriate experiments with pigeons an inner ear effect would fail to occur. Instead of the stria vascularis, the pigeon possesses a somewhat different epithelia in the cochlea (tegmentum vasculosum) and its DC potential is considerably lower than that in animals [Schmidt and Fernandez, 1962; Necker, 1970]. The first evidence that considerable differences in the effect of the EA between the species exist was presented recently by Wit and Bleeker [1982] and Schermuly et al. [1983]. These authors found that after the application of EA and furosemide in the pigeon, the CAP was only slightly affected. Corresponding morphological and functional investigations have not yet been carried out on pigeons.

Should it be, that loop diuretics do not affect the inner ear of the pigeon, i.e. the cochlea and the vestibular organ, this reaction would correspond to the reaction of the guinea pig's vestibular organ. For humans, the destruction of the vestibular apparatus has only been described in the case of sublethal doses [Arnold et al., 1981], so that the question arises of whether or not a dose-effect relationship exists. Consequently one must also ask if intoxication with loop diuretics actually causes 'ototoxicity' of the ear if alterations in the labyrinth are to be interpreted as unspecific effects within the general framework of toxicity on the total organism.

The question of dose dependency for the vestibular organ was investigated in guinea pigs by Kusakari et al. [1979]. In the experiments of these authors, an effect could only be achieved with high doses. Dose-effect curves, similar to those obtained by the authors above, were also determined by Morgenstern et al. [1981] for another diuretic (ozolinon). In appropriate experiments with guinea pigs, it was shown that the relation of diuretic to ototoxic effect was many times higher for ozolinon than for EA or furosemide. In order to determine whether the effect of the EA in the pigeon labyrinth was actually 'ototoxic' or not, it was necessary to examine the cochlea of the pigeon after different doses of EA in analogy to investigations on the vestibular organ of the guinea pig. In this way one could collect reference points for a delineation between specific and unspecific effects.

The mechanism of effect of the loop diuretics in the inner ear is presently still unclear. Due to the similarities of the secretory cells in the inner ear and those in the kidney, it was assumed that they functioned with a similar mechanism, especially because the diuretic and the ototoxic effects usually began at the same time. It could also be shown, that in the kidney the renal perfusion and the glomerular filtration rate are somewhat lowered by loop diuretics [Greven et al., 1978; Greven and Heidenreich, 1978]. Furthermore, this category of diuretics suppresses the tubular chloride reabsorption more than the sodium reabsorption and allows the potassium secretion to increase. At the same time, the urinary pH is shifted toward a neutral value and the tubular secretion of paraaminohippuric acid (PAH) is suppressed.

The potassium and sodium concentrations after EA administration parallels those in the kidney. Whereas – as mentioned – the chloride transport is mainly inhibited in the kidney, nothing is known of a possible change of this electrolyte in the inner ear. An investigation of this ion may give insight into the actual mode of action of EA in the inner ear.

Owing to the introduction of the stereoisomeres of the diuretic drug ozolinon, it became possible to increase knowledge of the mode of action of loop diuretics in the ear. Ozolinon is a diuretic which, similarly to furosemide and EA, also inhibits the electrolyte reabsorption in the ascending loop of Henle of the kidney. Due to an asymmetric carbon atom, there are two optical isomeres of this substance [Satzinger et al., 1978]. It has been proven that only the left-turning form is active as a diuretic (*l*-ozolinon); the right-turning form (*d*-ozolinon) does not lead to a diuresis. It is not yet known whether comparable reactions can also be expected in the inner ear. Therefore, the influence of the right-turning as well as the left-turning form of ozolinon on the DC potential of the guinea pig was investigated. In this manner an experimental instrument is created with which one can relate the effect of the substance on the inner ear to the known 'double-tracked' mode of action in the kidney.

The diuretically inactive ozolinon isomere is able to inhibit the diuretic effect of furosemide. The right-turning form, with an intravenous dosage of 10 mg/kg body weight, was shown to antagonize completely the diuretic effect of 1 mg/kg body weight of furosemide [Greven and Heidenreich, 1980]. It is not yet known if this effect also occurs in the ear.

Investigations so far have shown that a verification of the term 'ototoxicity' for the loop diuretics seems to be indicated when one compares their effect on the ear with results of experiments on the kidney in regard to their mode of action, their effect on cochlea and semicircular canals and their dose dependency. There is, however, another aspect of the discussed substances which deserves special interest. As mentioned initially, these substances can change the production and absorption of the endolymph. This is of importance, since presently a generally accepted concept as to the production and resorption of endolymph does not exist. Since the

investigations of Shambaugh [1907] and Guild [1927], it is generally
assumed that the stria vascularis is the main production site of the
endolymph in the cochlea. Von Békésy [1952] was the first to discover the
unusually high potential of $+80$ mV in the endolymph. Tasaki et al. [1954]
could confirm these results. At approximately the same time, Smith et al.
[1954] first determined the electrolyte concentrations in the endolymph
space. The above authors found a high-potassium and a low-sodium
content which corresponded to the concentrations of both ions in the
intracellular space. Further measurements [Citron and Exley, 1957; Johnstone et al., 1963] confirmed these results. The functional meaning of this
uniquely high potential, as well as of the high-potassium concentration in
the cochlear endolymph, is presently still unclear.

Therefore, in the mid-1950s, the stria vascularis became the center of
attraction for electron microscope investigations [Engström et al., 1955;
Smith, 1957; Naftalin and Harrison, 1958; Hilding, 1965]. Significant
findings of the above-named authors were a three-layered structure of the
stria formed by superficial marginal cells, intermediate cells, and underlying
basal cells. The morphological picture with numerous mitochondria in the
marginal cells, a surface enlargement in the basal area caused by numerous
cytoplasmatic villi, a clearly developed Golgi apparatus, and superficial
microvilli indicated in analogy to epithelia in other organs (kidney, pancreas, choreoid plexus), a central role within the electrolyte and water
transport. Kimura and Schuknecht [1970] have supported these characteristics of the stria vascularis in the guinea pig through similar ultrastructural
findings in human petrous bones.

After EA application, the previously mentioned drastic changes of the
DC potential (-40 mV) occurred in conjunction with an interstitial edema
of the stria vascularis. In 1974, Sellick and Johnstone additionally demonstrated that the DC potential significantly decreased by EA, could be
elevated to -20 mV by subsequent anoxia. This effect could also be
achieved by oubain (strophantin). On the basis of these experiments and
the equally well-known changes of the sodium and potassium concentration
by EA and oubain application, Vosteen [1976] developed a still valid
concept, that there are most likely three forces, all dependent on each
another, which may be held responsible for the electrolyte movement across
the walls of the endolymph tubing: (1) an electropositive potassium pump
that may be blocked by EA, as well as (2) an electronegative sodium-potas-
sium exchange pump that may be blocked by oubain, and (3) an electronegative, passive potassium diffusion towards the perilymph, with a
concomitant sodium diffusion from the perilymph into the endo-lymph,
which always lowers the DC potential into the negative range when both
other active pumps fail to function as a result of anoxia.

From a comparison of morphological and functional findings after EA administration in different regions of the endolymph space, potentially new conclusions may be drawn. Currently, the term 'endolymph production' is most commonly used. However, because of the different potentials in the cochlea and ampulla in mammals ($+80$ versus $+4$ mV), we ought suppose as to whether or not the endolymph in the various labyrinthine regions is produced by different mechanisms. A comparison of the findings resulting from the application of EA in guinea pigs and pigeons should hopefully give further information about the normal regulation of the endolymph.

In summary, the experiments presented here have the following goals: (1) to clarify the current application of the term ototoxicity, and (2) through the application of loop diuretics, taking into consideration differences in species, to examine the prevailing concepts of the endolymph production in the cochlea as to their validity for the vestibular apparatus and to pursue the question of whether or not the endolymph production obeys the same principles in all labyrinthine regions.

The clarification of these questions was approached by means of animal experiments (guinea pigs, pigeons). As representative loop diuretics, EA and the stereoisomeres of the ozolinon were employed. To obtain a morphological parameter of the diuretic effect, light microscopic, transmission electron microscopic and scanning electron microscopic investigations were carried out. At the same time, the corresponding measurement of the endolymphatic equilibrium potential and the potassium and sodium concentrations in the endolymph space were used as parameters of the functional influence of the tested substances.

2. Material and Methods

2.1. Experimental Animals and Preparation

The morpholigical and electrophysiological investigations were carried out on a total of 64 pigmented guinea pigs and 47 pigeons (*Columba domestica*). The body weight of these animals varied between 230 and 440 g.

The animals were anesthetized by intraperitoneal administration of 25% urethane. Further preparation was performed on a warming pad according to individual body temperature (guinea pig 37 °C, pigeon 41 °C). The tracheotomy was performed via a longitudinal cutaneous incision in the supine position. This procedure was completed with the insertion and the fixation of an adequately fitting PVC tube in the tracheostoma. The animal was placed flat on its abdomen. The head was secured with an especially constructed apparatus. Only animals with a positive Preyer reflex were used.

For the guinea pigs, the further procedures were as follows: preparation and opening of the bulla from ventral with exposition of the cochlea and the horizontal semicircular ampulla.

In the case of the pigeons, whose cochlea forms a straight tube, the region of the oval gap was approached laterally and exposed at the base of the cochlea. Access to the semicircular canals and ampulla was achieved from a somewhat more cranial-lateral approach. For this purpose, the osseous lamellae of the cranium had to be removed so that all the semicircular canals could be readily accessive.

2.2. Loop Diuretics

EA (hydromedin, formula $C_{13}H_{12}C_{12}O_4$) and ozolinon (formula $C_{10}K_{15}N_2O_3S$) were used as loop diuretics. From the structural formulas presented in figure 1, it can be seen that the ozolinon has an asymmetric carbon atom and, therefore, two optical isomeres of this substance exist. Both the left-turning form (l-ozolinon) as well as the right-turning form (d-ozolinon) were tested as to their effect on the inner ear. For EA, dosages of 60, 80 and 100 mg/kg body weight were used. Ozolinon was applied in dosages of 400 mg/kg body weight and 1000 mg/kg body weight.

A diuretic effect of the loop diuretics was assumed with spontaneous urination. Quantitative and qualitative measurements were not recorded. All substances were administered intravenously. For the purpose of better handling during later repositioning of the animals, a well-fitting plastic catheter was inserted into the jugular vein before further preparation. The injection time was usually 3 min. However, for the application of sublethal doses (see results), the duration of injection sometimes had to be extended to 10 min.

2.3. Tissue Preparation

Light Microscope. The fixation of the tissue of the guinea pigs was achieved by a local microperfusion of 2.5% glutaraldehyde with the help of a micropipette in the endolymph space after extraction of the stapes. After subsequent decapitation, the petrous bones were removed and again submersed in 2.5% glutaraldehyde with cacolydate buffer 0.1 mol for 24 h.

The extraction of the pigeons' cochleae followed decapitation and partial prefixation. Ampulla and semicircular canals were directly removed as skinny preparations without surrounding bone because of their easy accessibility. After a rinsing in cacodylate buffer, the preparations were finally fixed by means of 1% osmium tetroxide (Merck Corp.) and buffer at ambient room temperature. After subsequent renewed rinsing in buffer, dehydration was carried out stepwise in the ascending alcohol series (50, 70, 90, 96%, twice pure alcohol). At this point of fixation, all tissues to be examined (tegmentum vasculosum of the pigeon, stria vascularis of the guinea pig, ampullae as well as semicircular canals in the guinea pigs) were also freed from their surrounding bony structures. The subsequent embedding, took place stepwise in pure propylene oxide (Merck Corp.), in a propylene oxide-epon-812 mixture (Serva Corp.), and finally in pure epon-812 in the form of a flat embedding. Polymerization was achieved in an oven at a temperature of 30 °C for 24 h, and immediately thereafter at 60 °C for 48 h. Before finishing this procedure, the position of the tissue had to be inspected, since only certain cutting angles allowed an exposure of the epithelia under discussion here. The blocks were trimmed under the on-light microscope by means of a razor blade, and then semithin cuts were produced by an ultramicrotome (Reichert Corp.). The thickness of the slices was approximately 1 μm. Thereafter, the slices were stained with methylene blue for light microscopic investigation.

Transmission Electron Microscope. Ultrathin slices (thickness of slices 300–850 Å) were prepared for the transmission electron microscope. These were mounted on copper nets (150 or 200 mesh, partially with formvar film) after a double contrasting with uranylacetate and lead citrate. A Zeiss (EM 9 S-2) was available for the electron microscopic investigation. The acceleration voltage was approximately 60 kV; the magnifying power was between 1,800 and 27,000×. The film material used was Agfa-Gevaert, Scientia, 7 × 7 cm.

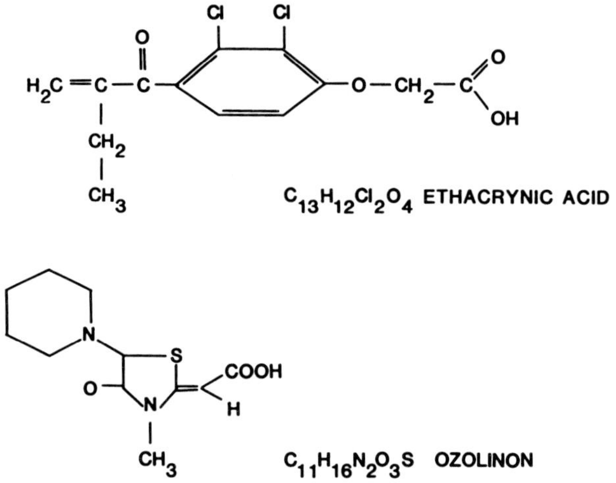

Fig. 1. Structure and net formula of the used loop diuretics EA and ozolinon.

Scanning Electron Microscopic Investigations. Until immersion into pure alcohol, the treatment of the preparations was the same as for the transmission electron microscope. The samples were then run through an ascending amylacetate series (Merck Corp.), with the individual steps being defined at 25, 50, 75% and 4 times 100% amylacetate. This was followed by 'critical point' drying, achieved over CO_2 (Polaron Corp.).

The micropreparation was carried out by means of microforceps and microhooks under a stereo-on light microscope. Then the preparations were mounted on bulbar-shaped supports with colloidal silver (Polaron Corp.). In a vacuum (0.05 Torr) they were subsequently 'sputtered' with gold, layer thickness 200–250 Å (Polaron Corp. with digital measurement of layer thickness). The scanning electron microscope investigations were performed with a device of the Contron Corp. (JSM-U3) with additional critical angle rectification at an acceleration voltage of 25 kV and magnifications between 135 and 15,000 ×. Ilford 120 FP4 was used as film material. The transmission and scanning electron microscope investigations were performed by Prof. Rosenbauer at the Institute for Anatomy of The University of Düsseldorf.

Problems Encountered During Tissue Preparation. Aside from following the generally known guidelines of this technique, the production of electron microscopic cuts also depends upon the skill in handling the preparations. A good fixation is a prerequisite for the quality of the samples. Principally, two modes of fixation are available: (a) a direct fixation of the tissue, and (b) the so-called total body fixation.

For our examinations of the secretory epithelia, we found that direct fixation via microperfusion was better than the total fixation. In the case of the latter, the fixation solution permeates the skinny endolymph tubing insufficiently because the skinny labyrinth is completely surrounded by bone [Wersäll, 1956; Anniko and Bagger-Sjöbäck, 1977]. This is also true for scanning electron microscope examinations. We noticed, however, that the stereocilia of the hair cells suffered from severe artefacts during the microperfusion. We attributed this phenomenon to clumping of the cupula and tectorial membrane, after application of glutaraldehyde with a poor subsequent fixation of the hair cells. Therefore, when examining the hair cells in the labyrinth, one should definitely use the total body fixation. The disadvantage of the local microperfusion can be attributed to 'turbulence' within the endolymph which can lead to superficial damage as well as to direct mechanical damage by contact with the tissue. We tried to avoid these disadvantages by the following methods: (1) Careful initial fixation of cochlea and ampulla via perilymph space. (2) Gradual exchanging of the endolymph for the fixation solution by means of a micropipette. (3) Opening of the endolymph tubing some distance from the organs to be examined (semicircular canal, oval window niche) instead of immediately above them.

The excision of skinny preparations of the pigeons offers the significant advantage that one avoids the subsequent decalcification and the artefacts related to it. Furthermore, the production of ultrathin cuts is subsequently easier. The disadvantage is to be seen in a potential mechanical irritation of the tissue secondary to the preparation. In order to avoid such damage, we found it helpful to first fix and solidify the tissue which was to be prepared. The excision of cochlear tissue is easier with prior decapitation and preparation of the excised petrous bone. However, even in these instances, an in vivo fixation by local microperfusion was performed.

2.4. Measurement of the Endolymphatic Potential, the
Potassium and Sodium Concentrations and Chloride Concentration

Construction of Electrodes. Double volume capillaries, the inner walls of which contain filaments (Hilgenberg Corp.) from Pyrex glass, served as raw material for the construction of the electrodes. Their outer diameter was 1.5 mm, the inner diameter 0.89 mm. They were cut to a length of 10 cm and cleaned with distilled water. After repeated rinsing with pure alcohol, they were dried at 200 °C for 2 h. With a capillary extension device (Albrecht Instruments Corp., Model GA-01286-A-B), they were pulled out under control by a light microscope with an appropriate scale to a tip diameter of 0.5 μm. For the measurement of the DC potential, this electrode was filled with a 2.7-mol KCl solution. The complete filling of the tip was also observed under the light microscope. A chlorinated silver wire was dipped into the KCl solution.

For the later measurement of the potassium and sodium concentrations in the endolymph space, double volume electrodes were used. After extension of the glass capillaries, the backward arm of the capillary was shortened in the way that the remaining piece measured approximately 3 cm from the sharp tip to the end of the capillary. The other arm was sealed with candle wax. Thereafter, the short arm was steam-coated with Silan for 45 s. After the wax-sealed part of the longer arm had been cut, the capillaries were heated up to 130 °C for 45 min so that the Silan steam could also reach the tip. The electrodes in the short 'Silanized' arm were then filled with the corresponding WPI ion exchanger. Then they were stored in a rack with their tips down for at least 24 h so that the ion exchanger could diffuse into the tip. The long 'not Silanized' arm of the electrode was filled with 160 ml KCl solution. This procedure was controlled under the light microscope. The short 'Silanized' arm of the potassium electrodes was filled with 160 mmol KCl solution; the sodium electrodes with 160 mmol NaCl solution. The tips of these electrodes were broken manually to a diameter of 2–5 μm. Both arms were filled again, free of air bubbles, with the above 160 mmol ion solutions. Hanging in an exsiccator, the bottom of which was filled with a 100-mmol potassium chloride and 160 mmol sodium chloride solution, respectively, so that the tips of the electrodes were submersed in the solution, the electrodes were stored in the refrigerator until calibration.

Calibration of Electrodes. Four different calibration solutions were prepared for the calibration of the potassium electrodes. For this purpose, KCl solutions with a molarity of

160, 80, 16 and 8 mmol were adjusted to a total osmolarity of 160 mmol by adding an adequate amount of NaCl. For the calibration of the sodium electrodes, six calibration solutions were needed (160, 80, 16, 8, 4 and 1 mmol NaCl solution). The larger number of calibration solutions for the sodium electrode calibration was necessary because the calibration graph curves in the lower range (ca. 1–8 mmol). For the sodium measurement in the scala media, the values are just in this range (about 6 mmol). It was necessary, therefore, to define this curve precisely.

A high-impedance voltage meter (WPI Corp., model F-223 A Dual-electrometer) served as a measuring instrument. It was hooked up to two polygraphs: one for the measurements of potassium and sodium (Rikadenki Corp.) and one for the endolymphatic potential measurements (Philips Corp.). Measurements took place in a Faraday cage (fig. 2).

The long arm of the electrode was then placed in a connecting piece that had been filled with 160 mmol KCl solution. A chlorinated silver wire was dipped into the short arm. The connecting piece as well as the silver wire were cabled up with the input and output of the measuring device. In this way, the long capillary arm with the KCl solution became the reference electrode and the short capillary arm with the corresponding ion exchanger became the active signal electrode.

Calibration was performed by immersing the electrodes into the descending series of calibration solutions. The 160-mmol KCl and NaCl solutions were again measured as a control. The potential differences of the individual solutions were registered by the graphs. The values measured were plotted on semilogarithmic paper for the determination of the calibration curve. The curve's bend in the lower range reflects the fact that a simultaneous registration of potassium ion had a visible effect of the measured sodium ion concentration.

The semilogarithmic plotting of the measured values is derived from the Nernst equation. The calibration solutions were kept at a temperature of 37 °C in a water bath provided with a thermostat. That was in order to minimize the influence of temperature, which is an important variable in the equation. At this temperature it can be concluded from the Nernst equation, that at a concentration ratio of 1:10 (e.g. 16 and 160 mmol), the potential differences should reach 61.5 mV. The electrodes used for the measurement reached values between 52 and 65 mV. The impedance values of the potassium electrodes were below $10^{10} \, \Omega$, and of the sodium electrodes in the range of 10^{10} and $10^{11} \, \Omega$. Calibrations were performed before and after the measurements as a control.

Measurement of the Endolymphatic Potential (Ductus cochlearis Potential). As described in section 1.1, a tracheotomy and canulation was performed on the anesthetized experimental animals on a heated operating pad under maintained spontaneous respiration. The rectal temperature, as measured by an electrical thermometer (Bailey Corp., model BAT 8), was plotted simultaneously. For the guinea pig, the bulla, as described above, was freed ventrally and then opened, thereby exposing the cochlea. For the pigeons, the region of the oval window slit, which includes the base of the cochlea, was prepared by a lateral approach. The exposition of the ampullae in guinea pigs and pigeons was achieved with the same approach as described under section 1.1 for the excision of the histological preparations. Under a light microscope, the osseous wall delineating the stria vascularis in the third winding, the tegmentum vasculosum, and the ampullar structures was penetrated, creating a bore hole of approximately 40–50 μm. By means of a micromanipulator, the glass electrode was inserted through this hole into the endolymphatic space. A chlorinated silver wire served as reference electrode which was advanced into the cervical musculature. Measurements were carried out with a potentiometer (Keithly Corp.), the input impedance of which was $10^{14} \, \Omega$. The liquid leaving the extracellular perilymphatic space at the prepared site served as reference voltage with a potential of 0 mV. The proper position of the electrode tip could be assessed by the potential difference between this liquid and the endolymphatic space.

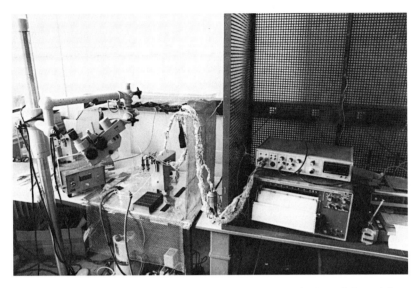

Fig. 2. Setting of the measurement equipment for the determination of the endolymphatic potential and the ion concentrations. Faraday cage with heatable operating table, calibration solutions, micromanipulator and microscope (left). High impedance potential measuring device with triplegraph (right).

The loop diuretics were administered intravenously via a catheter previously inserted into the jugular vein (section 2.2). The alterations of the DC potential were recorded by means of the compensatory polygraph. In order to exclude electrical field disturbances, the complete measuring equipment was placed in a Faraday cage. At the end of the recording, for the control purposes, the potential of the extracellular space was reset again in order to exclude a possible zero drift of the electrode.

For the measurement of the ion concentrations, adequately calibrated double volume electrodes like those described above were employed. By means of the micromanipulator, they were advanced into the endolymphatic space through the established bore hole, as explained above. The proper position of the electrode tip could be verified by the respective positive potential in the endolymph.

The measurements of the endolymphatic potential as well as of the ion concentrations could be recorded simultaneously. After the recording, the ion concentrations were determined by transferring the values from the potential graphs onto the previously prepared calibration graphs.

Criticism of the Method. The use of ion-sensitive electrodes for measurement of potassium and sodium activity has definite advantages over other methods of measuring concentrations (i.e. glass electrodes, flame photometer). The measurement is taken directly without intervention of chemical reactions. This results in saving time and avoiding many possible mistakes which are caused by complicated procedures. At the same time, continuous measurements are possible, whereas with other procedures, measurements can only be made at certain definite times. The simultaneous measurements of the endolymphatic potential and the ion concentrations made it possible to know in which part of the endolymph region the ions were being recorded. In using methods in which endolymph is extracted by suction (i.e. flame photometry) one cannot help getting endolymph from different regions in the extract, even when only small amounts are taken. Our method allowed us to measure the ion concentration at a defined site in the endolymphatic space. Even the measurements with glass electrodes do not fill the requirement of concurrent measurements of ion concentration and DC potential used here, since a simultaneous measurement with the glass electrode method is impossible. Finally, ion-sensitive microelectrodes have the advantage of having a very tiny tip diameter. This reduces damage to the surrounding tissue to a minimum and practically avoids the contamination of the endolymph.

On the other hand, the method used here contains two possible sources of error: (a) errors which may arise from the use of the microelectrodes themselves, and (b) errors which may arise from the application of the Nernst equation.

The incomplete specificity of the microelectrodes for a certain ion is a problem which belongs to the first group. However, regarding the effect of the potassium ions on the sodium measurement, this disadvantage may be corrected readily by a particularly precise calibration of the electrodes for the spectrum of the lower ion concentrations. A further error can be caused by the very high impedance of the measuring electrode (below 10^{10} for potassium electrodes, 10^{10} to $10^{11}\,\Omega$ for sodium electrodes). This makes it possible for electric fields to interfere with potential measurement. The interference, however, is avoidable by placing the measurement equipment in a Faraday cage. A final source of error is the so-called 'junction potential', a potential that results from diffusion between electrolytes of different composition, in this case between ion exchangers and endolymph, which is measured in potential. Since the 'junction potential' also occurs during the calibration, it has been disregarded.

Among the errors which arise from the application of the Nernst equation is the effect of temperature on the measurement. The problem is caused by the temperature difference between calibration solutions and the labyrinthine liquid. Although the calibration solutions were set at a temperature of 37 °C (guinea pig) and 41 °C (pigeon), and the body temperatures of the animals were kept as constant as possible by a heating pad, due to the unavoidable rapid cooling of the experimental animals under anesthesia, an exact temperature adjustment could not always be achieved.

The influence of the temperature on the measured values is clearly understandable when one considers the fact that 1 °C equals a potential change of 1 mV and, therefore, for sodium measurements in the range of 10 mmol a change of 0.5 mmol or for potassium measurement in the range of 160 mmol a change of 4 mmol.

Another error, however, occurred only during the measurement of the potassium concentrations. The reason is that, in the Nernst equation, the logarithm of the ratio of the ion concentrations has to be calculated. Thereby, a potential difference of a few mV corresponds to a constantly increasing concentration difference, especially for higher concentrations. Since higher concentrations are only measured for the potassium ion, the sodium measurements and, consequently, the sodium conduction and permeabilities derived therefrom remain unaffected. Additional errors possibly arising from the variance of the measuring electrodes were reduced to a minimum because the mode of construction was the same for all electrodes. The electrodes had to comply with the following requirements: (1) tip diameter between 2 and 5 μm; (2) tolerated potential difference of 52–56 mV for a concentration ratio of 1:10 for the potassium electrodes and 55–62 mV for the sodium electrodes; (3) approximate congruence of the calibration curves before and after the measurements.

3. Results

3.1. Morphological Findings in the Cochlea of the Guinea Pig Following Application of Ethacrynic Acid

After an EA dose of 60 mg/kg body weight, the stria vascularis was examined under the electron microscope at intervals of 0.5, 1, 2, and 3 h. A slight interstitial edema between the intermediate cells was first observed 30 min after the initiation of the experiment, and was most pronounced after 60 min. In all animals we examined, we found an extreme expansion of the intercellular space between the intermediate cells (fig. 3). The intermediate cells shriveled simultaneously in the same extreme manner. In some slides a significant increase of vesicles and vacuoles in the cytoplasm of the intermediate cells became obvious (fig. 4). A similar increased formation of vacuoles occurred within the marginal cells (fig. 5); a vacuolization of the mitochondria could also be seen occasionally. The rough endoplasmatic reticulum was distended at certain points. On the surface of the marginal cells, pinocytotic vesicles sometimes appeared. The zonula occludens and adherens between the marginal cells remained closed; the basal cells did not appear to be altered. Among the animals we examined, only a discrete swelling of the marginal cells could be observed.

The interstitial edema between the intermediate cells was essentially gone 3 h after administration of EA. In order to investigate the functional changes in the cochlea that go along with the strial edema, we examined the DC potential as well as the potassium and sodium concentrations in the endolympth after application of EA.

3.2. DC Potential, Potassium and Sodium Concentration in the Cochlea of the Guinea Pig Following Application of Ethacrynic Acid

From an initial value of $+80$ mV, the DC potential declined rapidly 8–10 min after injection of 60 mg/kg body weight EA, reaching a value of -40 mV within 10 min. Twenty minutes after this decline, there occurred again a sharp rise of the potential. After 40 min, it reached a value of about $+20$ mV. The further increase of the potential was much more gradual. In the 2 h post-injection period which we set arbitrarily, the potential eventually stabilized at $+40$ mV (fig. 6).

Somewhat later than the DC potential (approximately 20 min), the potassium concentration declined continuously during an hour, from 160 mmol to approximately 95 mmol. Thereafter, it slowly started to rise again. Two hours after application of EA, it was noticed a recovery to 130 mmol, but still had not reached the original concentration level.

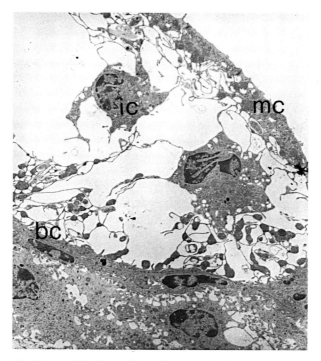

Fig. 3. Interstitial edema of the stria vascularis of the guinea pig 1 h after 60 mg/kg body weight EA. The intercellular space between the intermediate cells is voluminous swollen, the intermediate cells themselves shrunk. Discrete swelling of the marginal cells with the zonula occludens and adherens being without change. The basal cellular layer is intact. mc = Marginal cell; ic = intermediate cell; bc = basal cell. EM. ×3,200

The sodium concentration increased parallel to, yet somewhat earlier than, the potassium concentration. Circa 40–50 min after EA administration, the sodium concentration reached a value of 30 mmol. Thereafter, it declined again. With 14 mmol 2 h after EA application, the sodium concentration had not yet reached the initial value (6.2 mmol).

In summary, the results of the above experiments showed that the stria vascularis responds morphologically to the EA administration with a specific interstitial edema, a phenomenon that was linked to a rapid decline of the DC potential and changes of the sodium and potassium concentrations of the endolymph. The next section deals with the question of whether or not similar alterations occur in the ampulla and semicircular canals.

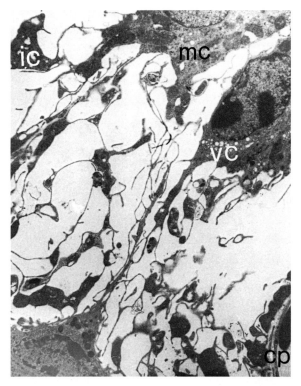

Fig. 4. Stria edema 1 h after EA administration in the guinea pig. The intermedaite cells containing pigment are severely shrunk. The marginal cells contain an increased number of small vesicles and vacuoles. mc = Marginal cell; vc = vacuole; ic = intermediate cell; cp = capillary. EM. ×4,800.

3.3. Morphological Findings in the Ampulla and the Semicircular Canal of the Guinea Pig Following Application of Ethacrynic Acid

In the apparatus of the semicircular canals there are various types of epithelia which are responsible for the regulation of the endolymph. For this reason we investigated the influence of EA on the dark cells, the cells of the planum semilunatum and the one-layered epithelium of the semicircular canal. All of these elements are involved in the above-mentioned function.

One hour after EA administration, there was only a discrete increase of the interstitial volume between the dark cells on the slope of the crista ampullaris. The assessment of an actual edema is made difficult, because between the dark cells of a control group which had not been given EA, one found a significant variance in the width of the interstitial space (fig. 7).

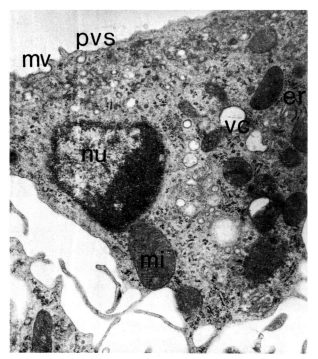

Fig. 5. Marginal cell 1 hr after 60 mg/kg body weight EA. Increased cytoplasmatic vesicle and vacuole formation. Superficially separation of a pinocytotic vesicle; vacuolization of a mitochondrium. Hydropic rough endoplasmatic reticulum. The cell nuclues without alterations. nu = Nucleus; mi = mitochondrium; er = endoplasmatic reticulum; vc = vacuole; pvs = pinocytotic vesicle; mv = microvilli. EM. ×8,800.

Furthermore, one could also observe a swelling of the mitochondria as well as protrusions of the cytoplasm in the endolymphatic space. The zonula adherens and occludens remained narrow. After EA application, there was also an increased vesicle formation, in particular in the apical region of the cytoplasm. As a peculiarity of the ampulla, we found among the dark cells a diffuse scattering of melanocytes containing large pigment deposits of melanin. After EA application, we had the impression that the melanocytes began to move, forming a tight chain underneath the dark cells. They also seemed to tend to nestle among the dark cells.

In the area of the cell cluster of the planum semilunatum on the lateral ampullar walls. EA application did not produce an interstitial edema. Occasionally, however, a vacuolization of the mitochondria and an increased number of multivesicular bodies and lysosomes could be found here (fig. 8).

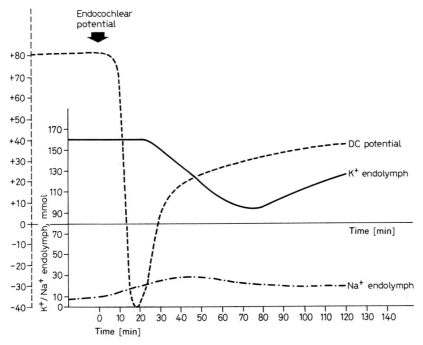

Fig. 6. The effect of 60 mg/kg body weight EA on the DC potential, the potassium and sodium concentrations in the endolymph of the guinea pig.

The one-layered cuboidal epithelium of the skinny semicircular canal also did not show any visible alteration under the electron microscope after application of EA (fig. 9). Unlike the cochlea, the epithelia in the ampulla showed only discrete morphological alterations after application of EA, so that we now had to examine the functional alterations in the endolymph space of the ampulla.

3.4. Endolymphatic Potential and Potassium and Sodium Concentrations in the Semicircular Canal of the Guinea Pig Following Application of Ethacrynic Acid

Due to the preparatory technique, the endolymphatic potential of the guinea pig was measured in the lumen close to the ampulla and not directly in the ampulla. For two reasons, however, one can assume that the initial potential in this region is the same as that in the ampulla itself. Firstly, the lumen is in the immediate vicinity of the ampulla and, secondly, we know that the endolymphatic potential on the opposite side of the ampulla, in

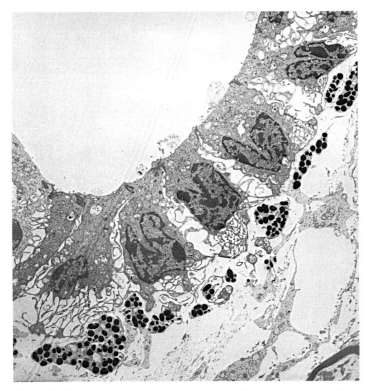

Fig. 7. Dark cells of the guinea pig 1 h after EA administration. Protrusions of cytoplasm into the endolymph space. Swollen mitochondria and invariably tight apical cell contacts besides a discrete interstitial accumulation of water, invariable cell nuclei. Tightly fitting chain of melanocytes. EM. ×3,550.

other words in the utriculus, is as in the ampulla, +4 mV [Sellick and Johnstone, 1974].

We found that the EA administration, the endolymphatic potential in the semicircular canal rose from an initial +4 mV very gradually to +6 mV within a period of 20 min and subsequently declined very slowly to −14 mV during a time period of 2 h (fig. 10). In the same time period, the potassium concentration declined only slightly (from 130 to 118 mmol). These values corresponded to a discrete increase of the sodium concentration from 32 to 40 mmol.

In the guinea pig, the effect of the EA in the vestibular region is significantly different from that in the cochlear area. In the electron microscope one sees discrete alterations which electrophysiologically correspond to a slight decrease of the endolymphatic potential and minor

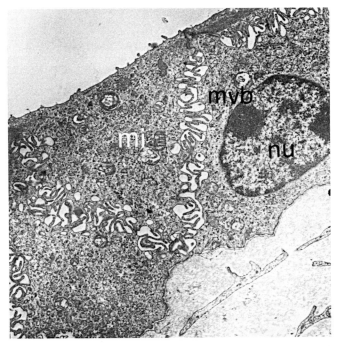

Fig. 8. Planum semilunatum 1 h after EA administration. No interstitial edema. The cell nuclei are unaltered. Rare vacuolization of mitochondria and multivesicular bodies. nu = Nucleus; mi = mitochondrium; mvb = multivesicular body, EM. × 8,400.

alterations of the electrolyte concentrations (potassium and sodium). In order to investigate this differing effect more precisely, we examined the effect of EA on the ampulla of the pigeon. It was first necessary for us to familiarize ourselves with the epithelial structures in the pigeon's ampulla, especially because no similar investigations have been published yet. For this purpose, in addition to the use of the light microscope and transmission electron microscope, the scanning electron miscroscope technique seemed to be the most appropriate method of investigation.

3.5. Scanning Electron Microscope Examinations of the Normal Structure of the Pigeon's Ampulla

In the pigeon, just as in the guinea pig, the ampullae of the horizontal and the posterior semicircular canals are located close together, i.e. they jointly end in the utricle (fig. 11). The ampulla of the vertical semicircular canal communicates with the utricle on the opposite side. In both, the posterior as well as the vertical ampullae, bilateral to the crista ampullaris,

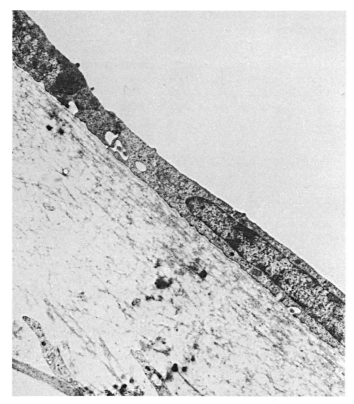

Fig. 9. Epithelium of semicircular canal 1 h after EA administration. There are no visible cellular alterations. EM. ×9,100.

we found the so-called eminentia cruciata. These are two protrusions which form a right angle to the crista ampullaris and are covered with secretory cells. Such structures could not be found in the horizontal ampulla.

In alternating sequence, light and dark cells appear on both sides of the eminentia cruciata. However, it was interesting to note that in the wedge region of this eminentia, only light cells could be seen. This peculiarity was found in all animals we examined (fig. 12). The dark cells showed abundant microvillar lining. In contrast, the light cells had very few microvilli and a somewhat centrally placed kinocilium (fig. 13). The surface showed small depressions and indentations, as seen in other secretory epithelia in the scanning electron microscope. The analysis of the transitional zone revealed hexagonal cells and alternately arranged light and dark cells. No differences could be seen between different types of light cells.

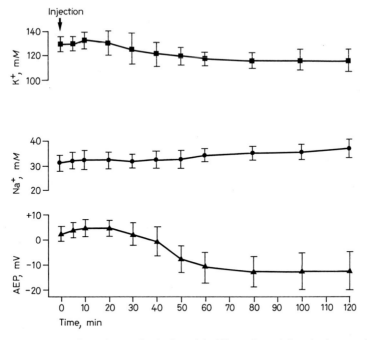

Fig. 10. The effect of 60 mg/kg body weight EA on the endolymphatic potential of the semicircular canal as well as the potassium and sodium concentrations in the semicircular canal of the guinea pig.

In the next section, the light microscopic and transmission electron microscopic peculiarities of the pigeon's ampulla will be dealt with in the discussion of the effect of EA applications.

3.6. Morphological Findings in the Ampulla of the Pigeon Following Application of Ethacrynic Acid

In the ampulla of the guinea pig, the administration of EA elicited discrete alterations in the dark cells only, most predominantly in the melanocytes. The interstitial edema, typical of that seen in the stria, did not appear. Consequently, the question arose, which morphological alterations of the pigeon's ampulla were caused by EA applications. In the slides which were examined 30 min after EA application, there were no alterations in the light or dark cells of the eminentia cruciata.

In contrast to the ampulla of the guinea pig, one can easily detect through the light microscope, the light and dark cells arranged in an alternating sequence, just as we had seen in the scanning electron microscope investigations (fig. 14). Sixty minutes after EA administration, the

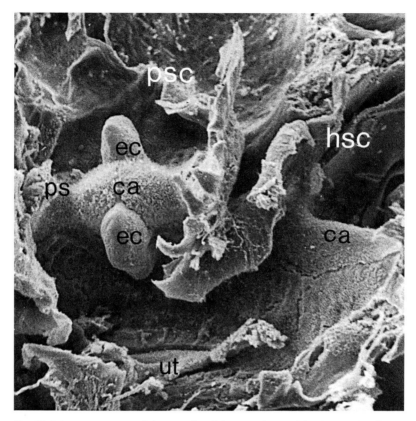

Fig. 11. Joint arrangement of the ampulla of the posterior semicircular canal (left) and the horizontal semicircular canal (right), which jointly end in the utricle (below). The cristae ampullares are covered with hair cells which have stereo- and kinocilia. The posterior ampulla of the semicircular canal is characterized by an eminentia cruciata, that is absent in the horizontal ampulla. On the lateral walls of the ampulla at the end of the crista ampullaris, the epithelia of the planum semilunatum are to be found. ca = Crista ampullaris; ec = eminentia cruciata; ut = utriculus; ps = planum semilunatum; psc = posterior semicircular canal; hsc = horizontal semicircular canal. REM. × 108.

intercellular gaps at the base of the dark cells appeared somewhat wider. However, similar to the guinea pig ampulla, there was a wide variance among the normal findings. Therefore, it was difficult to attribute this change to the effect of EA. In order slides, when seen under the light microscope, the light cells appeared to be swollen 60 min after EA administration (fig. 15), but there did not appear to by any definite interstitial edema.

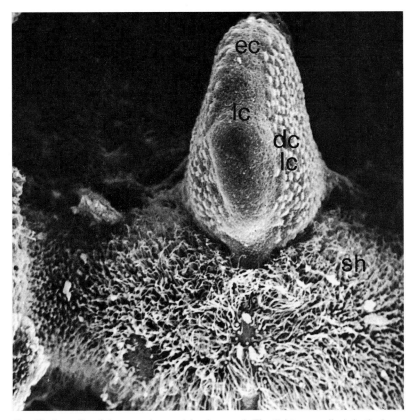

Fig. 12. Ampulla of the posterior semicircular canal. The Crista ampullaris in the lower part of the picture is covered with sensory hairs. With an angle of 90° the eminentia cruciata raises above. The alternating arrangement of microvilli-lined dark cells with bilaterally interspersed light cells may be well identified. On the ridge of the eminentia cruciata there are only light cells with a scarce microvillar lining. sh = Sensory hair; dc = dark cell; lc = light cell; ec = eminentia cruciata. REM. × 360.

During the scanning electron microscope investigations, we could see that the ridge of the eminentia cruciata was completely covered by light cells. It was interesting that we observed a change only in this region, which appeared in the light microscope as a clear interstitial edema 60 min after EA administration (fig. 16). However, we observed a swelling in the neighboring light cells which were dispersed with dark cells.

Three hours after EA application, the interstitial edema between the light cells in the ridge zone of the eminentia cruciata was no longer present. Worthy of note was the different coloring of the cytoplasma of these light cells. Some of them appeared quite dark (fig. 17).

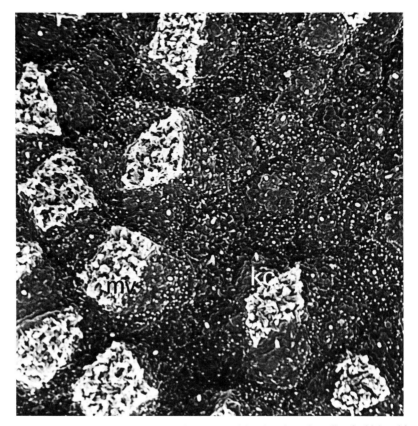

Fig. 13. Eminentia cruciata. Section from a transitional region, the cells of which, with a microvilli lining, may still be seen in the left part of the picture. The right margin of the picture shows the location of transition into the ridge of the eminentia cruciata. The light cells carry a longer kinocilium. The surface of these cells is lightly folded. A difference between the light cells arranged besides the dark cells and the light cells arranged separately cannot be established. REM. ×4,800.

Under the electron microscope, the interstitial edema between the light cells could be observed more closely. Thirty minutes after EA administration, there was an initial interstitial edema. The zonula occludens and adherens were tightly connected with each other. The remaining cell connections (desmosomes) in the region of the later cell membrane were also still intact. Here the edema developed mainly above and below the individual desmosomes (fig. 18).

Sixty minutes after the effect of EA, resolution of the desmosoma cell junctions also occurred. The volume of the interstitial space increased

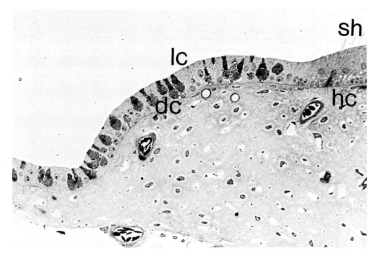

Fig. 14. Transitional zone with light and dark cells in the pigeon's ampulla 60 min after EA administration of 60 mg/kg body weight. Only very scarcely the intercellular gaps at the base of the dark cells appear to be somewhat widened. Between the light and the dark cells there is no interstitial edema. The cell contacts are closed; at the right margin of the picture one identifies the hair cells with their sensory hairs. lc = Light cell; dc = dark cell; hc = hair cell; sh = sensory hair. LM. × 200.

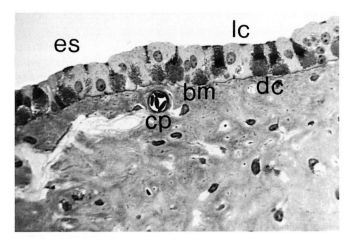

Fig. 15. Clear and dark cells of the slope of the eminentia cruciata 60 min after EA administration. No interstitial edema. Slight tendency towards a swelling of the light cells. The cell nuclei are unchanged, the intercellular gaps between the cytoplasmatic extensions of the dark cells do not show any increase of their volume. lc = Light cell; dc = dark cell; bm = basal membrane; cp = capillary; es = endolymph space. LM. × 320.

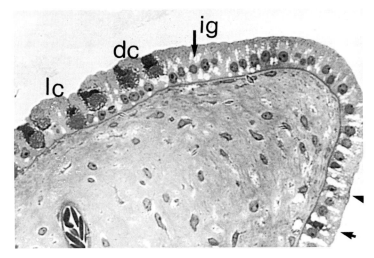

Fig. 16. Transverse cross-section of the eminentia cruciata 60 min after EA administration. The widening of the intercellular gaps (marked by arrows) is clearly evident only in the region of the tightly packed columnar-like light cells in the ridge zone. A significant swelling of the cytoplasm is observable in the neighbouring light cells, interspersed with dark cells. The intercellular gaps between the cytoplasmatic extensions of the dark cells are only slightly widened. lc = Light cell; dc = dark cell; ig = intercellular gap. LM. ×200.

significantly. Zonula occludens and adherens remained unchanged, however. Furthermore, an increased vesicle formation could be noticed within the light cells (fig. 19). The basal membrane covered by semidesmosomes was intact. The cell nucleus was not eroded. With stronger magnification, the increased number of vesicles could be identified as stimulation of the Golgi apparatus. Numerous vesicles were extruded from this complex.

The endoplasmatic reticulum appeared massively swollen. In some instances, a bursting of its membrane allowed the ribosomes to disperse themselves freely in the cytoplasm. The cristae mitochondriales showed signs of destruction. Concurrently, deposits of vacuoles could be seen in the mitochondria themselves.

On inspection of the dark cells, a slight though not very pronounced increase in the number of vesicles was visible. The vesicle increase in the light cells which were surrounded by dark cells was much more pronounced. The mitochondria of the dark cells were mostly intact. The endoplasmatic reticulum was not swollen in the same way as in the light cells. However, a scattering of free ribosomes and an increased activity of the Golgi apparatus was also seen here. In the region of the dark cells, no significant interstitial edema could be seen, even under the electron microscope.

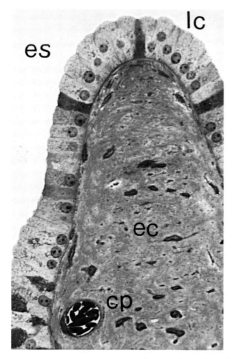

Fig. 17. Transverse cross-section of the eminentia cruciata 3 h after EA administration. The interstitial edema in the ridge zone between the light cells is no longer present. A variably strong staining of the cytoplasm of these cells is clearly detectable. lc = light cell; ec = eminentia cruciata; cp = capillary; es = endolymph space. LM. ×320.

Three hours after EA administration, the vesicles and vacuoles in most slides had joined together in some instances with dark granula to form so-called multivesicular bodies. At certain points one had the impression, that large vesicles and vacuoles moved towards the granula as if they wanted to be assimilated by them (fig. 20–26).

We also examined the effect of EA on the cell cluster of the planum semilunatum on the later ampullar walls which are also considered to be secretory cells. No morphological alterations were seen either with the light microscope or with the electron microscope (fig. 27, 28).

Our next step was to examine the functional alterations which accompany the swollen light cells, and the interstitial edema between the light cells of the eminentia cruciata in the endolymphatic space. For this we measured the endolymphatic potential and the potassium concentration in the ampulla of the pigeon after EA administration.

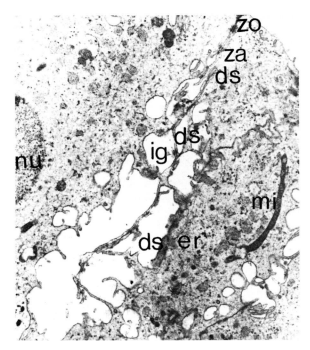

Fig. 18. Light cells of the ridge zone of the eminentia cruciata, 30 min after EA administration. Beginning widening of the intercellular gaps, with the desmosomal junctions however being largely intact. The superficial cell contacts with the zonula occludens and adherens are invariably tight. Swelling of the endoplasmatic reticulum. Unremarkable longitudinally stretched mitochondria. zo = Zonula occludens; za = adherens; ds = desmosome; ig = intercellular gap; nu = nucleus; mi = mitochondrium; er = endoplasmatic reticulum. EM. × 7,650.

3.7. Endolymphatic Potential and Potassium Concentration in the Ampulla of the Pigeon Following Application of Ethacrynic Acid

In a preliminary pilot study, we first measured the normal endolymphatic potential in the ampulla of the pigeon. We registered a value of 7.1 mV with a standard deviation of 0.5. At the same time, the mean of the potassium concentration was 166.0 mmol (fig. 29).

After administering EA in a dose of 60 mg/kg body weight, during the first 20 min after injection a minimal increase of the potential from 7.1 to 8.5 mV occurred. Forty minutes after injection, the initial potential of 7.1 mV was attained again and remained stable for the next 2 h. After EA administration, the potassium concentration declined to a value of 140 mmol within 30 min. Thereafter, in the course of 2 h it gradually attained the initial value of 160 mmol.

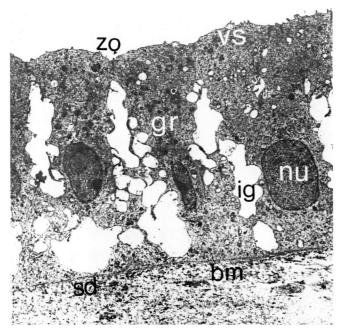

Fig. 19. Light cells of the eminentia cruciata zone 60 min after EA administration. Clear widening of the intercellular gaps. The desmosomal cell contacts are largely torn, the zonulae occludens and adherens though are still tight. Increased formation of vesicles, which head towards the surface at some locations, in the supranuclear cytoplasm. Cell nucleus and basilar membrane are unaltered. zo = Zonula occludens; vs = vesicle; gr = granula; ig = intercellular gap; nu = nucleus; bm = basilar membrane; sd = semidesmosome. EM. × 2,870.

Although there was no decrease of the endolymphatic potential in the pigeon's ampulla after EA administration, the initial increase still needs to be interpreted in the light of our findings. The simultaneous decrease of the potassium concentration, which was small yet pronounced, indicated that the potential cannot be directly related to the potassium concentration.

Aside from the interstitial edema in a circumscribed epithelia zone of the eminentia cruciata in the pigeon, one observed only unspecific morphological alterations in the sense of a swelling of the light cells. These changes had no functional effect on the endolymphatic potential in the ampulla.

In order to investigate whether EA was also nontoxic in the cochlea – an assumption suggested by the experiments of Schermuly et al. [1983] – we then determined the morphological and functional effects of EA by measuring the DC potential and the potassium concentration in the pigeon's cochlea. At this point, it should be stated again that the pigeon does not have a stria vascularis but rather secretory epithelia on the roof of

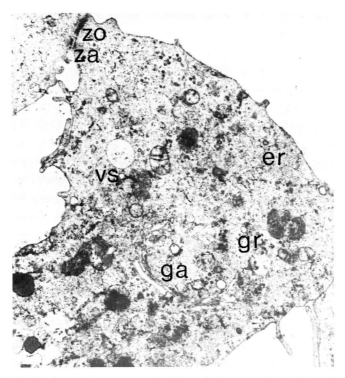

Fig. 20. Supranuclear aspect of a light cell from the ridge of the eminentia cruciata 60 min after administration. Significant widening of the intercellular gaps. The desmosomal contacts are interrupted whereas the zonulae occludens and adherens are invariably tight. Busy activity of the Golgi apparatus with increased extrusion of vesicles. Activity of the granulae which fuse at some locations and join to form larger particles. ga = Golgi apparatus; gr = granula; vs = vesicle; zo = zonula occludens; za = zonula adherens; er = endoplasmatic reticulum. EM. × 12,000.

the cochlea (tegmentum vasculosum) which are equated with the light and dark cells of the ampulla in the literature (fig. 29a). Therefore, we first examined by scanning electron microscope inspection whether or not this equation is valid.

3.8. Scanning Electron Microscope Examinations of the Normal Structure of the Pigeon's Cochlea

The cells of the tegmentum vasculosum villously protrude into the endolymph space from the roof of the ductus cochlearis. These villi stand at an angle of 90° to the longitudinal axis of the cochlea. A certain symmetry may be observed as the villi often overlap like a zipper in the

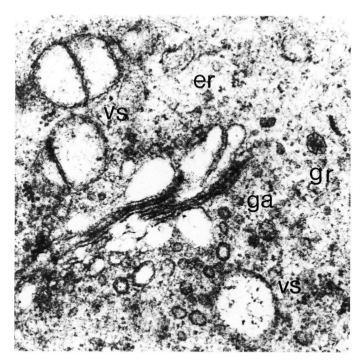

Fig. 21. Light cells 60 min after EA administration. Pronounced activity of the Golgi apparatus with extrusion of multiple vesicles. Widening of endoplasmatic reticulum lined with ribosomes. ga = Golgi apparatus; vs = vesicle; er = endoplasmatic reticulum; gr = granula. EM. × 43,000.

midline (fig. 30). The surface is formed by a checkerboard-like arrangement of alternating cells of different character with mostly hexagonal surfaces. In accordance with the same structural principle as in the ampulla of the pigeon, the dark cells here are also characterized by an abundance of microvilli. In contrast, aside from a scattering of microvilli, the light cells usually have a kinocilium. Often it is in the center. At times, however, it may also be found at the margin (fig. 31). The light cells often show a surface characterized by indentations that could suggest a secretory function. Cytoplasmatic protrusions are observable here and there.

3.9. Morphological Findings in the Pigeon's Cochlea Following Application of Ethacrynic Acid

Unlike that of the guinea pig cochlea, the structural difference of the secretoric epithelia in the cochlea of the pigeon can be seen clearly on slides using the light microscope (fig. 32). Instead of the stria vascularis of the

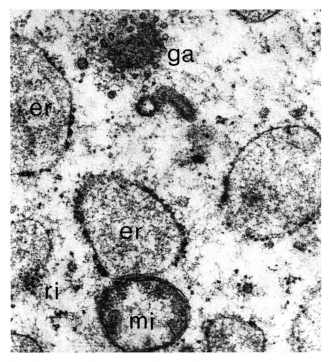

Fig. 22. Supranuclear part of a light cell from the ridge zone of the eminentia cruciata 60 min after EA administration. Extreme widening of the endoplasmatic reticulum the membrane of which may rupture and partially the ribosomes may freely spread in the cytoplasm. Transversely cut Golgi complex. The mitochondria are partially vacuolized and contact the endoplasmatic reticulum. er = Endoplasmatic reticulum; ga = Golgi apparatus; mi = mitochondria; ri = ribosome. EM. × 43,000.

guinea pig with its three-layered structure, the tegmentum vasculosum and, similarly, the epithelia of the eminentia cruciata and the transitional zone in the ampulla of the pigeon are composed of alternating light and dark cells.

After application of 60 mg/kg body weight of EA, there was no discernible interstitial edema between these different cells under the light microscope. With stronger magnification, one was able to see a swelling in some of the light cells only. The cytoplasma of these cells appeared disseminated and quite light, especially in the area around the nucleus. The darker cells showed no signs of change (fig. 33).

Thirty minutes after EA administration, a slight hydrops of the light cells was visible in the electron microscope (fig. 34). This swelling resulted in a cap-like protrusion of the light cells' surface into the endolymph space, a finding that was most pronounced 60 min after EA application (fig. 35).

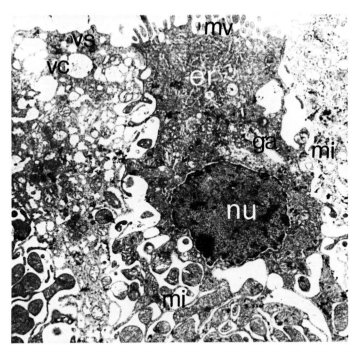

Fig. 23. Light and dark cells eminentia cruciata 60 min after EA administration. Significant increase of the formation of vesicles in the zone of the light cells which head towards the surface. In the vicinity massive vacuoles. Discrete widening of the intercellular gaps between light and dark cells. No signs of nuclear damage. The mitochondria in the area of the cytoplasmatic folds of the dark cells do not appear altered. Busy activity of the Golgi complex in the supranuclear part of the dark cell. The superficial cell contacts are tight. vs = Vesicle; vc = vacuole; nu = nucleus; mi = mitochondrium; er = endoplasmatic reticulum; ga = Golgi apparatus; mv = microvilli. EM. ×7,650.

The zonulae occludentes and adherentes remained impermeable. The cell organelles, especially the endoplasmatic reticulum and the Golgi apparatus, did not exhibit any significant alterations. An interstitial edema could not be noticed. In the area of the dark cells, one had the impression that there was an increased vesicle formation apically, although this differed significantly from cell to cell. There was also no edema between the plasmatic protrusions of the dark cells. Unfolding of these gaps spaces, observed in a few solitary locations, must be considered as a normal form variant.

In all slides, the swelling of the light cells vanished no later than 3 h after EA administration (fig. 36, 37). The cell surfaces were smooth again and exhibited some single indentations as well as beginning vesicle tie-offs (micropinocytotic vesicle).

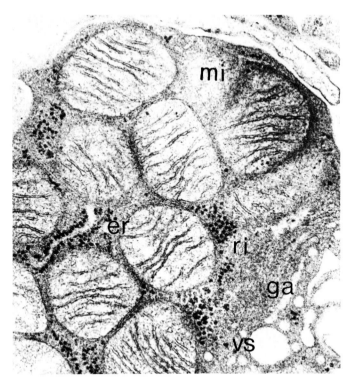

Fig. 24. Dark cells 60 min after EA administration. Unchanged mitochondrial structure. Busy activity of the Golgi apparatus with vesicular extrusions. The endoplasmatic reticulum is lined with ribosomes which partially begin to loose contact and are freely spread in the cytoplasm. mi = Mitochondrium; er = endoplasmatic reticulum; ri = ribosome; ga = Golgi apparatus; vs = vesicle. EM. ×43,000.

In summary, it may be concluded from these experiments that EA does not lead to an interstitial edema between the individual secretory cells in the pigeon's cochlea. The next step was to determine which functional alterations were elicited in the pigeon's cochlea by the administration of EA.

3.10. DC Potential and Potassium Concentration in the Cochlea of the Pigeon Following Application of Ethacrynic Acid

In the first series of experiments we began by determining the DC potential of the pigeon cochlea in normal animals in order to compare our values with those in the literature. We registered a DC potential of 13.8 mV with a measuring electrode which had been placed next to the oval recess in the endolymph compartment. The potassium concentration was measured simultaneously at an average of 165.0 mmol. The position of the tip

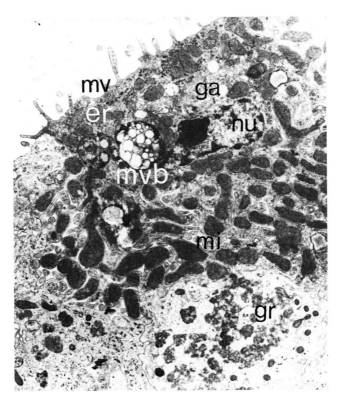

Fig. 25. Dark cells 3 h after EA administration. Dark granula and vesicles have joined to form a large multivesicular body. At the right lower margin of the picture, pigmented granula with scarce formation of membranes in the sense of lysosomal activity. mv = Microvilli; er = endoplasmatic reticulum; ga = Golgi apparatus; nu = nucleus; mvb = multivesicular body; mi = mitochondrium; gr = granula. EM. × 44,700.

of the electrode can be seen in figure 38. From this schematic drawing, one can also see the anatomical difference between the cochlea of the pigeon and that of the guinea pig. In comparison to the cochlea of mammals, the most pronounced difference is that of the straight construction of the 'snail' and the rudimentary construction of the scala vestibuli which only exhibits two bulges (fossa vestibuli and cisterna vestibuli).

Ten minutes after slow injection (3 min) of 60 mg/kg body weight of EA, there was a slight increase in the DC potential to a value of 14.5 mV. Thereafter, a slight decrease of the DC potential occurred. It declined to 12 mV, somewhat below the initial value. One hundred minutes after EA administration, the initial value of 13.8 mV was reached again (fig. 39).

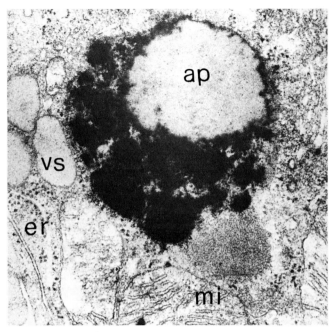

Fig. 26. Light cell from the ridge zone of the eminentia cruciata, appearing electron-dense, 3 h after EA administration. Dark granulae and vesicles form an autophagosome which may be also interpreted as lysosome. The vesicle at the left margin of the picture seek tight contact with it. ap = Autophagosome; vs = vesicle; er = endoplasmatic reticulum; mi = mitochondrium. EM. × 43,000.

In the same experimental protocol, the potassium declined slightly to a value of 160 mmol after approximately 30 min, remaining stable from there on. Taking into account the previously mentioned different possibilities for methodical errors, one may conclude that after administration of EA in a dose of 60 mg/kg body weight, the DC potential in the cochlea of the pigeon as well as the potassium concentration did not change.

During the measurements of the DC potential in the cochlea of the pigeon, it had become apparent that EA had to be administered intravenously over a time period of at least 3 min. More rapid injections lead to significant tachycardias of the experimental animals. Furthermore, despite slow 3-min injections, 2 animals died within 50–70 min after EA administration. Up to this point, however, neither of these animals had shown any changes in their DC potentials or potassium concentrations.

This observation led to the assumption that, for the pigeon, the effective dose of EA is very near to the lethal dose. In order to clarify this hypothesis, we worked in a subsequent series with different doses of EA

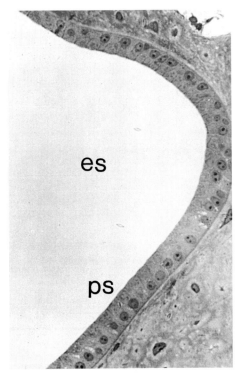

Fig. 27. Columnar-like cells of the planum semilunatum 60 min after EA administration. The cells are arranged in tight conjunction. The cell nuclei are unaltered. The slight distortion of the intercellular contacts to be observed at some locations is not significantly changed in comparison with the control group. ps = planum semilunatum; es = endolymph space. LM. × 200.

and measured the DC potential and potassium concentration in the endolymph of the pigeon's cochlea. The issues to be clarified were: (1) whether or not higher doses of EA led to any sort of a decrease in the DC potential, and (2) whether or not this decrease in the DC potential can still be considered as a specific effect on the inner ear.

3.11. Dose-Dependent Effect of Ethacrynic Acid on the DC
Potential and the Potassium Concentration in the Cochlea of the Pigeon

In preliminary studies with doses of 80 mg/kg body weight EA, it was found that all experimental animals died within 15–30 min after an injection given over a period of 3 min. Therefore, we extended the injection periods to 10 min for this series of experiments. But, despite this precaution, in only half of the animals we were able to record the DC potential

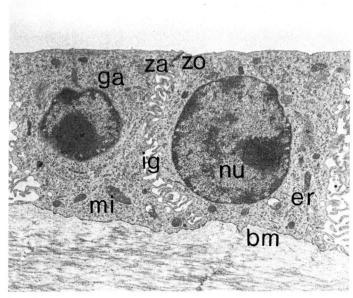

Fig. 28. Planum semilunatum 60 min after EA administration. Normally developed fingerlike toothing of this cell cluster without signs of the interstitial edema. The zonulae occludens and adherens are tightly closed. Pronounced Golgi apparatus and endoplasmatic reticulum. The cell nucleus is not changed. zo = Zonula occludens; za = zonula adherens; ga = Golgi apparatus; ig = intercellular gap; nu = nucleus; mi = mitochondrium; er = endoplasmatic reticulum; bm = basilar membrane. EM. × 14,400.

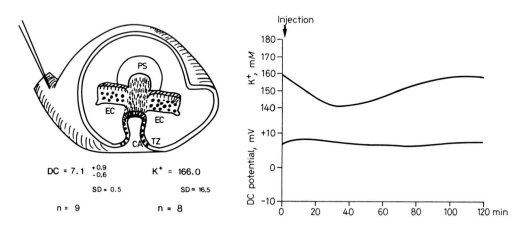

Fig. 29. a Schematic arrangement of the different ampullar structures with placement of the electrode tip. ca = Crista ampullaris; ec = eminentia cruciata; ps = planum semilunatum; tz = transitional zone. *b* The effect of EA (60 mg/kg body weight) on the endolymphatic potential (bottom curve) and the potassium concentration (upper curve) in the ampulla of the pigeon.

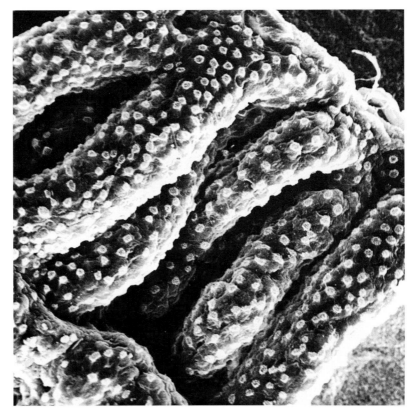

Fig. 30. Normal appearance of the tegmentum vasculosum. Villous arrangement of the tegmentum folds which overlap zip-like in the midline. Variable cell formations with mostly hexagonal surface delimitations. Alternating arrangement of cells which are abundantly lined by microvilli (dark cells) and cells which show a smooth surface (light cells). REM. × 480.

throughout a time period of 2 h. The other half of the experimental animals died of EΛ intoxication before the designated recording period was over. Figure 40 presents an example of a typical curve of the DC potential and potassium concentration after application of 80 mg/kg body weight EA.

After an initially slow decrease of the DC potential to a value of +10 mV over a time period of approximately 20 min, a somewhat faster decrease to −10 mV occurred after 50 min. A gradual recovery took place after ca. 2 h and ended at a value of −3 mV. The initial 13.8 mV was not reached. Under this dosage, parallel to the decrease of the DC potential, there was a decline in the potassium concentration after 40 min from 165 to

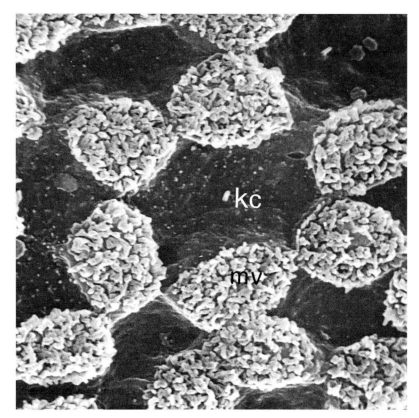

Fig. 31. Normal finding of the tegmentum vasculosum. Clearly visible cells with a lining of microvilli and interspersed cells with smooth surfaces. Here are scarcely scattered smaller microvilli. In the center of the picture a centrally arranged kinocilium of a light cell, as well as at the upper right margin of the picture. The surface of these cells is characterized by indentations as well as excavations at some locations (left margin of the picture). mv = Microvilli; kc = kinocilium. REM. ×7,200.

145 mmol, including a slight initial increase. Recovery set in far more slowly. However, after 2 h the initial value was attained again.

We increased the dose in 3 pigeons to 100 mg/kg body weight EA, with an injection period of 10 min. With this dose we observed a decrease of the DC potential to −28 mV within 15–25 min. All 3 tests animals died immediately thereafter. Prior to death, the potassium concentration had dropped below a value of 140 mmol. Even slower injections (over 15 min) could not avert the lethal outcome with these high doses.

From these experiments, in which we increased dosage and slowed injection rates, we concluded that the change of the DC potential, as

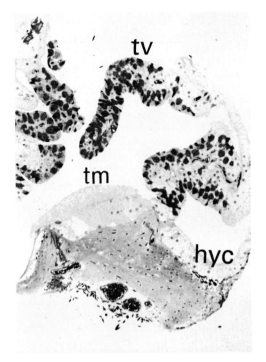

Fig. 32. Cross-section through the cochlea of the pigeon 60 min after EA administration. Unchanged arrangement of alternating light and dark cells which villously protrude into the endolymph space from the roof. No interstitial edema. tv = Tegmentum vasculosum; hyc = hyaline cells; tm = tectorial membrane. LM. × 80.

observed with a dose of 80 mg/kg body weight, must not be interpreted as a specific effect on the inner ear but rather as an expression of the overall toxic effect on the entire organism.

3.12. Chloride Concentration in the Cochlear Endolymph of the Guinea Pig Following Application of Ethacrynic Acid

As mentioned at the beginning, until now it had been assumed that the manner in which loop diuretics affected the inner ear was similar to that in the kidney. Because it is known that loop diuretics in the kidney reduce tubular chloride reabsorption, besides inhibiting sodium reabsorption and increasing potassium secretion, we investigated the influence of EA on the chloride concentration in the endolymph of the guinea pig.

The normal chloride concentration in the cochlear endolymph of the guinea pig is 119 mmol. After injection of 60 mg/kg body weight EA, we found a slight initial increase of this concentration to 122 mmol, with a

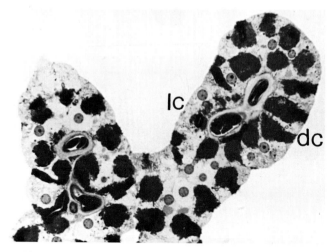

Fig. 33. Tegmentum vasculosum 60 min after EA administration. Partial hydrops of the light cells. The cytoplasm of these cells appears broken up and perinuclearly clearly lighter. The dark cells are unchanged, the basal cytoplasmatic extensions stand tightly packed and lack an interstitial edema. Both light and dark cells are in contact with the capillaries below the basilar membrane. lc = Light cells; dc = dark cells. LM. × 320.

drop to the initial value immediately thereafter. The chloride concentration did not change further during the course of the measurements. The simultaneously recorded decrease of the DC potential from $+80\,mV$ to $-40\,mV$ was also reproduced in this experimental setting. It corresponded to the values we had found earlier during the simultaneous measurement of the potassium and sodium concentrations (fig. 41).

3.13. DC Potential and Potassium Concentration in the Cochlea of the Guinea Pig Following Application of l-Ozolinon

With respect to perfusion, alterations of the sodium, potassium and chloride concentrations and the effect on the PAH secretion in the kidney, similar changes have been reported after administration of EA and furosemide on the one hand and ozolinon on the other. In order to assess the effect of loop diuretics and their mode of action in the inner ear, we examined the DC potentials and potassium concentrations in guinea pigs after administration of *l*-ozolinon, using the measurements described below.

After administration of 400 mg/kg body weight ozolinon, a rapid drop in the DC potential occurred with a subsequent recovery phase similar to that observed in the case of EA. At a dose of 100 mg/kg body weight, an equally rapid decline of the DC potential could be noticed. However, we

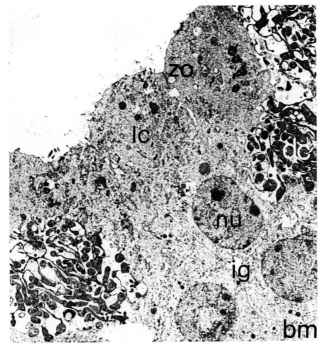

Fig. 34. Tegmentum vasculosum with light and dark cells 30 min after EA administration. Slight hydrops of the light cells with protrusion of the surface into the endolymphatic space. The apically located cell junctions as well as the basilar membrane were intact, the cell organelles were without any alterations. The interstitial spaces between the plasmatic foldings of the dark cells appeared somewhat widened although similar pictures were also seen of normal epithelia. lc = Light cell; nu = nucleus; zo = zonula occludens; ig = intercellular gap; bm = basilar membrane. EM. ×2,880.

saw a much slower and incomplete recovery of the potential as compared with the reaction after the dose of 400 mg/kg body weight ozolinon. A potential of merely +30 mV was obtained approximately 2 h after ozolinon administration.

In contrast to the EA experiments, even with higher doses of 1,000 mg/kg body weight ozolinon, a rapid drop of the DC potential occurred without a concurrent change of the potassium concentration in the endolymphatic space (fig. 42).

A dose of 60 mg/kg body weight EA produced a decrease in potassium concentration along with a drop in the DC potential. Among other changes, the morphological correlate of these functional alterations consisted of a swelling of the marginal cells. Therefore, we used the scanning electron microscope to see, if the different effects of EA and ozolinon on the

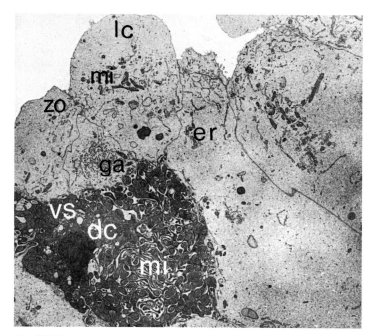

Fig. 35. Tegmentum vasculosum 60 min after EA administration. Maximal swelling of the light cells with cap like protrusion of the surface. The zonulae occludentes were also tight here. No interstitial edema, busy activity of the Golgi apparatus. Increased vesicle formation in the apical parts of the dark cells. The interstitial space between the cytoplasmatic foldings of the dark cells is not widened, the mitochondria normally configurated. lc = Light cell; mi = mitochondrium; zo = zonula occludens; er = endoplasmatic reticulum; ga = Golgi apparatus; dc = dark cell; vs = vesicle. EM. ×2,880.

potassium concentration correspond to different morphological changes in the marginal cells.

3.14. Scanning Electron Microscope Findings in the
Cochlea of the Guinea Pig Following Application of l-Ozolinon

Scanning electron microscope investigations of the marginal cells of the stria vascularis after administration of *l*-ozolinon demonstrated that only a slight swelling of the marginal cells occurred when a dose of 1,000 mg/kg body weight was administered. This substance simultaneously depressed the DC potential quickly without changing the potassium concentration in the endolymphatic space. Only with a higher dose of 1,500 mg/kg body weight did a more significant swelling of the marginal cells occur (fig. 43).

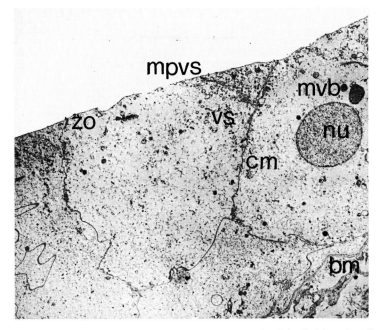

Fig. 36. Clear cells of the tegmentum vasculosum 3 h after EA administration. Complete resolution of the swelling resulting from EA. No interstitial edema. The surface of the light cells was characterized by small indentations as well as beginning tie-offs in the sense of micropinocytotic vesicles. Unremarkable cell junctions. Large cytoplasmatic inclusions of different electrondensity (multivesicular bodies). mpvs = Micropinocytotic vesicle; zo = zonula occludens; vs = vesicle; cm = cell membrane; mvb = multivesticular body; nu = nucleus; bm = basilar membrane. EM. ×2,880.

3.15. DC Potential in the Cochlea of the Guinea Pig
Following Application of d-Ozolinon

We examined the effect of *d*-ozolinon on the DC potential of the cochlea of the guinea pig at the same dosage (1,000 mg/kg body weight) since it had been demonstrated, that the right-turning form of the ozolinon did not have any diuretic effect in the kidney. We found, that *d*-ozolinon at this dosage did not cause a decrease of the DC potential. In simultaneous morphological controls we saw no changes resembling an interstitial edema as had been observed after EA (fig. 44). Since it is known, that the preadministration of *d*-ozolinon has an antagonizing effect on the diuretic effect of furosemide and EA in the kidney, we tried to find out, if a similar mode of action also exists in the inner ear.

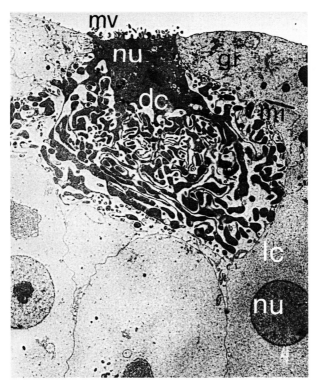

Fig. 37. Tegmentum vasculosum 3 h after application of ethacrynic acid. The light cells are only slightly swollen. Large, dark cytoplasmic inclusions in the light cells with normal appearance of cell organelles. The basal plasma folds of the dark cells exhibit a normal configuration. The volume of the interstitia in this area conforms to the scope of variation seen in normal specimens, so that one can conclude there is no interstitial edema here. mv = Microvilli; dc = dark cell; lc = light cell; m_i = mitochondria; nu = nucleus; gr = granula.

3.16. The Combined Effect of d-*Ozolinon and Ethacrynic Acid on the DC Potential in the Cochlea of the Guinea Pig*

d-Ozolinon was first injected intravenously at a dosage of 1,000 mg/kg body weight. A change in the DC potential over a time interval of more than 1 h was registered. We could observe only a minimal change of this potential to a value of ca. 70 mV. When the same animal was subsequently given EA at a dosage of 60 mg/kg body weight, a rapid decrease of the DC potential to a value of -10 mV occurred within 15 min. In summary, it may be concluded from this study that, unlike in the kidney, the antagonizing effect of *d*-ozolinon on the mode of action of EA cannot be applied to the stria vascularis in any case.

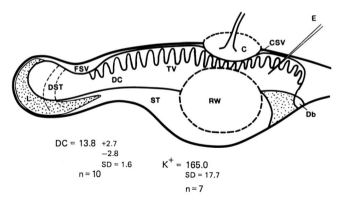

DC = 13.8 +2.7
            −2.8
        SD = 1.6 K^+ = 165.0
    n = 10   SD = 17.7
                            n = 7

Fig. 38. Schematic sagittal cut through the pigeon cochlea showing the position of the tip of the electrode. c = Columella; rw = round window; tv = tegmentum vasculosum; dc = ductus cochlearis; st = scala tympani; l = lagena; fsv = fossa scala vestibuli; csv = cisterna scala vestibuli; dst = ductus scala tympani; db = ductus brevis.

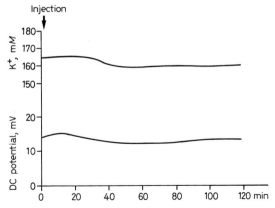

Fig. 39. The effect of EA (60 mg/kg body weight) in the pigeon's cochlea. DC potential (bottom curve), potassium concentration (upper curve).

4. Discussion

Research of the inner ear received important impulses through the clinical observation of deafness in connection with tuberculosis patients. The term ototoxicity was coined for tuberculostatica by morphological and animal experimental studies in which the target of destruction in the inner ear could be identified as damage to the outer hair cells of the organ of Corti. The functional correlate of this damage is a decrease of the summary action potential and of the cochlear microphonics. Due to the direct

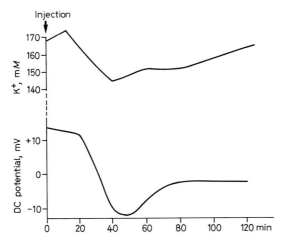

Fig. 40. The effect of EA (80 mg/kg body weight) in the cochlea of the pigeon. DC potential (bottom curve), potassium concentration (upper curve).

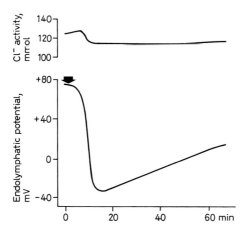

Fig. 41. The effect of EA (60 mg/kg body weight) on the DC potential and the chloride concentration in the guinea pig's endolymph.

damage of the hair cells by this group of aminoglycosides, it was not surprising that the functional impairments in the inner ear were irreversible. This could be confirmed in animal tests.

With the introduction of loop diuretics in dehydration therapy, similar manifestations of inner ear damage occurred. Most of these were reversible, and mainly affected the cochlea [Maher and Schreiner, 1965; Schneider and Becker, 1966; Vargish et al., 1970; Mathog et al., 1970; Schwarz et al., 1970;

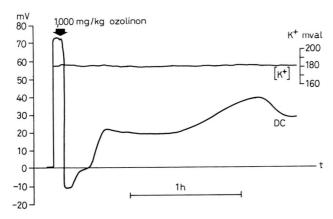

Fig. 42. The effect of *l*-ozolinon (1,000 mg/kg body weight) on the DC potential and the potassium concentration in the cochlear endolymph in the guinea pig.

Matz, 1976]. In analogy to the aminoglycosides, this side effect of the loop diuretics was also called ototoxic.

The particular conditions that existed among the patients who suffered from a hearing deficit after the administration of loop diuretics was the first evidence that an assumed ototoxicity of the loop diuretics cannot be compared to the ototoxicity of aminoglycosides. Contrary to the aminoglycoside antibiotics, hearing deficits after administration of loop diuretics only occurred when: (1) these substances had been given at an extremely high dosage, and (2) the consequences of a cumulative effect in the organism, e.g. uremia, were apparent clinically [Matz and Naunton, 1968].

These correlations could also be proven experimentally in anuric guinea pigs [McCurdy and McCormick, 1974]. To us the joint term ototoxicity for these different substances (aminoglycosides and loop diuretics) did not appear to be justified. The probability of side effects of drugs on other organs arises with increasing doses, like e.g. in the inner ear. For the aminoglycosides this dose is in the upper range, though still within the therapeutic range of these substances [Kurz and Neumann, 1977].

A completely different situation exists for loop diuretics. Their effective dose in humans is 0.5–1.0 mg/kg body weight. 50–100 mg/die as a daily dosis are also considered sufficient for the attainment of a forced diuresis. The producer recommends a maximum dose of 400-mg loop diuretics/die as this dosage is at the upper limit of the therapeutic range and an improvement of the effect is not to be expected by higher doses. From the clinical publications of untoward effects on the inner ear, it can be seen that in

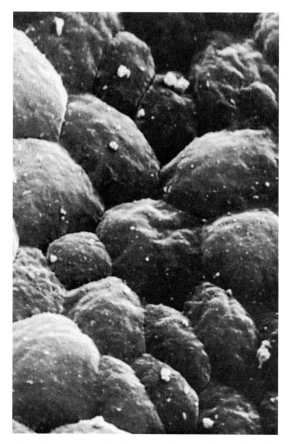

Fig. 43. Marginal cells 1 h after administration of *l*-ozolinon (1,500 mg/kg). The marginal cells are swollen and protrude cap-like into the endolymphe space. The surface of the swollen cells is sporadically characterized by tie-offs and indentations. REM. ×4,800.

those cases of hearing impairments following administration of loop diuretics this dose was always far exceeded. Comparing this clinical experience with experimental investigations on animals with inner ear damages, one sees a good correlation. A functional impairment of the guinea pig's inner ear performance is achieved only at doses of 40 mg/kg body weight, i.e. at doses which are approximately 6–8 times higher than those which should not be exceeded in order to take advantage of the maximal effect [Bosher, 1980].

    In summary, the conclusion has to be drawn from these toxicological considerations, that a special organ toxicity of the loop diuretics, as implied

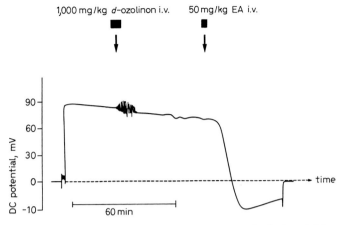

Fig. 44. The combined effect of d-ozolinon (1,000 mg/kg body weight) and EA (60 mg/kg body weight) on the DC potential in the endolymph of the guinea pig.

by the term 'ototoxicity', is only valid in a very limited sense, because it can only be achieved by extremely high doses.

The ototoxic characteristics of aminoglycosides have to be regarded differently in comparison with those of loop diuretics. This documented a potentiated effect on the inner ear when both substances were administered simultaneously. Duvall and Quick [1969] had reported a potentiated inner ear effect when streptomycin, gentamycin and kanamycin were administered together with loop diuretics. Similar findings were also reported by other authors [Brummer et al., 1975; Mathog and Capps, 1977; Nakai, 1971; Ohtani, 1978]. Notable in this context is Falk's [1972] publication, which states that the administration of loop diuretics significantly augments the degree of hair cell damage due to noise.

The potentiated inner ear damage caused by the drugs discussed here suggested a different mode of action in the ear. Quick and Duvall [1970] were the first to discover this mechanism. From a series of experiments it became clear, that the main site of destruction of the loop diuretics in the inner ear is the stria vascularis [Nakai, 1971; Bosher et al., 1973; Brummet at al., 1977; Arnold et al., 1978; Anniko and Sarkady, 1978; Bosher, 1979, 1980]. In contrast to hair cell damage after aminoglycoside administration, there is an interstitial edema of the inter-mediate cells as well as a hydrops of the marginal cells after loop diuretics. These alterations correspond functionally with a rapid decrease of the endolymphatic potential from +80 mV to −40 mV during 10–15 min. At the same time, the potassium concentration dropped and the sodium concentration increased in the endolymph. These alterations are morphologically as well as functionally reversible, so that the animal experimental results represent the clinical picture of predominantly reversible hearing impairments in humans. Unlike the aminoglycoside antibiotics, the loop diuretics do not change the DC potential. As mentioned, the hair cell damages here functionally correlate with a drop in the cochlear microphonics and the summary action potential.

In this study we examined once again this known effect of the loop diuretics on the stria vascularis. This procedure seemed to be necessary in order to demonstrate the accurate reproducibility of the described alterations as well as to examine the method.

Under the electron microscope we found an interstitial edema of the intermediate cells. These alterations were most evident after 1 h. Three hours after EA administration the edema had resolved substantially. At the same time there was a slight swelling of the marginal cells without destruction of surface cell contacts (zonulae adherens and occludens). Functionally, the DC potential had dropped from $+80\,mV$ to $-40\,mV$ within 18 min. After 2 h of drug effect, the potential had recovered to a value of $+40\,mV$. The potassium concentration in the endolymph dropped somewhat more slowly. A value of 95 mmol was reached 70–80 min after EA administration. After 2 h we measured 130 mmol for potassium. During the same interval the sodium concentration had increased from 6.5 to 32 mmol after 40–50 min and after 2 h had again reached a value of 20 mmol.

These alterations comply with the literature data, thereby proving that the electron microscope technique as well as the use of double volume ion sensitive microelectrodes in the manner in which we employed them produce reliable and reproducible results.

In the literature, subtle differences regarding the time sequence of the morphological and functional alterations are also reported. These, most likely, are caused by the use of different methods. For example, the decline of the DC potential after EA, was reported in the range of 8–18 min. In unpublished pilot tests we could trace these time differences to different modes in the administration of the loop diuretics (i.v. or i.p.). The delayed effect on the stria vascularis is probably caused by the delayed resorption after intraperitoneal administration.

Therefore, based on these experiments, the term 'ototoxicity' has a limited validity in terms of loop diuretics. In contrast to the aminoglycoside antibiotics, the target site here is the stria vascularis. Morphologically, a transient interstitial edema is seen and reversible functional alterations caused by declining DC potentials and electrolyte changes also occur. Within the therapeutic range, only doses much higher than those of the aminoglycosides caused reversible hearing damage. The ototoxicity of the aminoglycosides can also be extended to include the vestibular portion because they can damage the hair cells of the crista ampullaris of the semicircular ampulla as well as those in the organ of Corti [Causse, 1949; Farrington et al., 1947; Spönglin, 1966; Wersäll et al., 1973]. We examined the EA effect on the ampulla and the semicircular canal in the guinea pig both morphologically and functionally because until now only fragmented results were presented by different authors [Sellick and Johnstone, 1974; Kusakari and Thalmann, 1976; Lim and Freilich, 1981; Hommerich, 1985].

In conclusion, we found no interstitial edema in the ampulla as seen under the electron microscope with the same dose (60 mg/kg body weight) which was used for the cochlea. Varying deposits of water in the interstitial space between the dark cells was interpreted as being a normal variation. Lim and Freilich [1981] had similar results. The authors interpreted the discrete edema as a result of different fixation methods. After pure osmium fixation there were no further interstitial widenings. Standardized electron microscope fixation with glutaraldehyde guaranteed comparability with stria vascularis results. Meyer zum Gottesberge-Orsulakova [1986] recently explained the hydrops of the light cells in the ampulla of the guinea pig as an EA effect. These morphological findings were discovered with the freeze cut technique without any means of fixation. The swelling of the light cells and an intracellular increase of the sodium concentration occurred 40 min after drug influence. The substitution of potassium-rich endolymph with a sodium-rich solution caused a similar swelling. The less prominent change in the light cells in the guinea pig ampulla will be taken up later in the discussion of the experimental results with the pigeon.

The absence of interstitial edema in the stria vascularis and of marked changes in the DC potential and of changes in the electrolyte concentrations in the ampulla are decisive criteria for defining a possible 'vestibular toxicity . In the labyrinth section we found only weak functional alterations after EA administration. After 30 min, the endolymphatic potential in the ampulla began to decrease very slowly and reached -14 mV after 2 h. The potassium concentration also decreased slightly from 130 to 118 mmol and the sodium concentration increased from 32 to 40 mmol within the same time period.

Our functional results correspond to the findings of Kusakari and Thalmann [1976]. These authors measured the endolymphatic potential in the ampulla of the guinea pig. They discovered that the potential did not change with a dose of 50 mg/kg body weight and decreased slightly with a dose of 70 mg/kg body weight to -6 mV after 2 h. Sellick and Johnstone [1974] also showed that the endolymphatic potential in the utricle of the guinea pig could not be influenced by a comparable EA dose. They could only produce a decrease of the potential by local injection into the endolymph space.

From these results of comparative experiments of the effect of loop diuretics on the stria vascularis and secreting epithelia in the mammal ampulla, one must conclude that these drugs are not 'ototoxic' in reference to the vestibular region. Therefore, this label must be modified because it is valid for damages to the cochlea, and then only under certain circumstances.

We examined the well-developed ampulla of the pigeon after EA to verify the missing vestibular ototoxicity in the labyrinth. There were no functional alterations of the endolymphatic potential. The native value of $+7.1$ mV compares well with the low values for the guinea pig ampulla. Initially we registered a temporary increase to $+8.5$ mV. To exclude EA as the cause of the potential changes, we injected experimentally an equal volume of NaCl intravenously. It also resulted in a slight initial potential increase. We attributed this 'injection effect' to the vascular volume increase.

The main morphological change in the ampulla of the pigeon was a swelling of the light cells. The circumscribed interstitial edema near the eminentia cruciata will be discussed later. As already mentioned, this interstitial edema probably was a side effect, a premise which is supported by the absence of functional alterations, as the applied EA dose did not cause a reduction of the endolymphatic potential in the ampulla.

With the same dose of EA, we obtained similar morphological results in the light cells of the cochlea of the pigeon. These alterations were most pronounced 1 h after drug injection and vanished after 3 h. The next question was whether or not the swollen light cells represented functional damage in the cochlea of the pigeon. Functional results gave the answer: the endolymphatic potential in the pigeon's cochlea remained unchanged during the 2 h following EA administration (60 mg/kg body weight). There was also no change in the potassium concentration in the endolymph. We concluded therefore, that, because of the lack of functional changes, the swelling of the light cells in the cochlea and ampulla of the pigeon does not represent a specific organ toxicity.

A similar effect was found on the light cells in the kidney [Richet and Hagège, 1975] and in the secretory epithelia of the salivary glands of the rat [Knauf and Sachs, 1980]. Richet and Hagège [1975] showed that the renal light cells are responsible for the resorption of sodium and the secretion of potassium. The dark cells secrete hydrogen and resorb potassium and are dependent on the acid-base metabolism. Kregenow [1977] described the swelling of light cells in different tissues as a general EA effect. The swelling coincided with an increase of the intracellular sodium concentration. In the regeneratory phase, the cells tended towards 'overcompensation', with shrinkage to a so-called minimal volume which represented 80% of the initial volume. The precise mechanism of this sodium increase is still unknown.

By using the freeze cut technique, as mentioned above, Meyer zum Gottesberge-Orsulakova [1986] could demonstrate swelling of the light cells in the ampulla of the guinea pig after EA. When we used the author's proposal (60 mg/kg body weight) we were not able to produce a functional impairment in the ampulla. Therefore, we interpreted the swelling of the light cells as a general effect of EA, as we did in the above-mentioned organs. Most likely, the swelling is a response to the sodium transport.

Using the electron microscope we also found changes of the cell organelles of the swollen cells in the cochlea of the pigeon. These were interpreted as response to their volume shifts in the context of their general cell function. The endoplasmatic reticulum is also considered by other authors to play a role in the volume regulation of the cell [McNight and Leaf, 1977; Civan, 1978]. Our experiments found further a scattering of vacuoles in the mitochondria. Various alterations on other cell organelles were also interpreted by us to be a generalized reaction by these cells in order to cope with 'toxic phenomena'. This includes the stimulation of the Golgi complex after EA administration, as well as the fusion of vesicles of different electron density to form so-called 'multivesicular bodies' in the regeneratory phase after drug influence. In other secretory epithelia (kidney and pancreas) these 'multivesicular bodies' also constitute in varying numbers the basic equipment of this cell type [Novikoff, 1963].

The alterations listed after EA administration, in particular in the light cells, are, in the ampulla of the guinea pig and the ampulla and cochlea of the pigeon, the result of the general characteristic of loop diuretics which is to impede the transport of electrolyte (sodium). In addition, one must consider a change of the membrane permeability for ions as another possibility. Considering this, the morphological alterations are not surprising. One cannot conclude from this evidence, however, that an 'ototoxicity' exists for this part of the labyrinth.

With comparable doses of EA producing functional as well as morphological changes in the cochlea of the guinea pig by affecting the stria vascularis, there were no ototoxic damages to either the cochlea or the ampulla of the pigeon. The importance of this finding is the fact that there were also no toxic morphological or functional consequences in the vestibular organ of the guinea pig. In contrast, as referred above, Kusakari and Thalmann [1976] measured a significant decrease of the endolymphatic potential in the ampulla of the pigeon with an increase of the dose. The authors concluded from this that loop diuretics may also be ototoxic for the vestibular portion. A repetition of these dose-related tests in the guinea pig ampulla did not appear to us to be necessary. We performed comparable tests on the pigeon cochlea in which no ototoxic effect had been seen by 'normal' doses. With 80 mg/kg body weight EA, a reduction of the endolymphatic potential to -12 mV occurred in the pigeon cochlea within 50 min. This took place much slower than in the guinea pig cochlea. After 2 h, a value of -4 mV was attained. The potassium concentration had dropped from 165 to 145 mmol after 40 min. The initial value of 160 mmol was almost regained after 2 h.

This dose of 80 mg/kg body weight, however, is close to the lethal dose. According to our tests, the LD_{50} of EA for the pigeon was between 80 and 100 mg/kg body weight. (With a dose of 100 mg/kg body weight, all pigeons were dead 30 min after injection.) At this time the endolymphatic potential was approximately -28 mV. The decrease of the endolymphatic potential after administration of loop diuretics, at least in the case of the pigeon, cannot be considered an ototoxic effect because the effect is only caused by sublethal doses and quite obviously represents an intoxication of the whole organism.

The species-specific LD_{50} values of the loop diuretics must be considered when one reviews the similar dose-dependent results in the guinea pig as seen by Kusakari and Thalmann [1976]. Compared to the pigeon, the LD_{50} is somewhat higher for EA in the guinea pig (around 200–220 mg/kg body weight). Consequently, a dose of 100 mg/kg body weight for this species already approaches the range of significant toxicity for the whole organism. Under toxological considerations, dose-dependent tests in the pigeon cochlea as well as our morphological and functional results from the vestibular guinea pig labyrinth, allow us to conclude that the ototoxicity of loop diuretics is closely related to the presence of the stria vascularis. Therefore, we propose the term 'striatoxic' to define the toxic effect of the loop diuretics as opposed to the 'ototoxic' effect of the aminoglycosides.

Before discussion of the specific sensitivity of the stria vascularis to the loop diuretics, we have to clarify two side effects caused by EA.

(1) Contrary to mammalians, the unprepared pigeon ampulla formed wall-like protuberances along the sides of the crista ampullaris. These formations were called 'septum transversum' by Retzius [1880], later 'septum cruciatum' by de Burlet [1935] and finally 'eminentia cruciata' by Dohlmann [1964]. Corresponding to the transitional zone of the mammalian ampulla, the eminentia cruciata is considered to be a significant surface increase of the secretory epithelia in the pigeon ampulla [Ishiyama et al., 1970; Igarashi and Yoshinobu, 1966; Ishiyama and Keels, 1971].

Under the scanning electron microscope, this eminentia cruciata was absent only in the ampulla of the horizontal semicircular canal of the pigeon. Lim [1971] however, saw a rudimentary form of the eminentia cruciata solely in the vertical ampulla of mouse and dog. Furthermore, in the pigeon there is a region at the roof of the eminentia cruciata that is exclusively covered by light cells. This peculiarity has not been noted before.

After EA administration there was reproducible interstitial edema between the light cells in this region. Approximately 3 h after EA administration, a varying cytoplasmatic staining of these light cells could be observed under the light microscope. Since the function of these epithelia is still unclear, this obviously EA-related effect in the pigeon's ampulla cannot be explained yet.

It is also difficult to assess whether these alterations can be connected with another surprising result from the pigeon ampulla. After EA application of 60 mg/kg body weight, the potassium concentration decreased from 166 to 140 mmol within 30 min. The initial value was reached again after 2 h. In contrast to the above-reported functional results from the guinea pig ampulla, the endolymphatic potential did not change here. Dohlmann and Boord [1965] reported a subsequent significant secretory activity, particularly in the light cells of the eminentia cruciata, in those experiments in which the cupula had been removed. The edema between the light cells and the concomitant potassium decline in the ampullar endolymph in the pigeon may be related to the ionic changes of the cupula. Further explanation of our results after EA administration may use these findings as a starting point.

(2) Stimulation of the melanocytes in the guinea pig ampulla was another side effect of EA administration. Since the experiments of Wolff [1931], we know that the pigment in the inner ear is melanin. Meyer zum Gottesberge-Orsulakova [1984, 1986] studied the melanin pigment in the inner ear with respect to the effect of EA on melanocytes. These effects were also confirmed by Lim and Freilich [1981]. Meyer zum Gottesberge-Orsulakova demonstrated a most pronounced decrease of the magnesium concentration in the melanocytes of the guinea pig ampulla after EA administration by means of the LAMMA (laser microprobe mass analysis) technique. Possibly the pigments in the inner ear are more involved in enzymatic reactions than assumed so far.

The loop diuretics are only toxic to the stria vascularis in the mammalian labyrinth. This effect is characterized functionally by a reversible decline of the DC potential. Because the interstitial edema and the electrolyte disturbances in the endolymph occurred simultaneoulsy, we explained the EA effect as a block of the postulated ion pumps and of enzymes potentially regulating these pumps. The classic publications by

Komnick and Komnick [1963] on the salt gland of fish emphasized the important participation of the interstitium in the electrolyte exchange with subsequent water shifts. Following the detection of the sodium-potassium-activated ATPase in the erythrocyte membrane [Post et al., 1960], scientific interest increased in this enzyme and the correlating electrolyte shifts [Skou, 1965]. The high ATPase content of the stria vascularis was often pointed out [Nakai and Hilding, 1966, 1967; Kuijpers, 1967, 1969; Matschinski and Thalmann, 1970]. Furthermore, the ATPase could be located under the electron microscope at the basolateral side of the intermediary cells [Ross et al., 1982; Kerr et al., Mees, 1983]. In the meantime, it is a well-known fact that EA acts indirectly on this enzyme in the stria vascularis [Konishi and Mendelssohn, 1970; Kuijpers and Wilbert, 1976; Paloheimo and Thalmann, 1977; Kusakari et al., 1978].

There are indications that EA significantly inhibits the adenylcyclase [Ahlström and Thalmann, 1975; Paloheimo and Thalmann, 1977; Bagger-Sjöbäck et al., 1980; Duvall et al., 1980; Anniko et al., 1981; Schacht, 1982]. Marumo and Mishinat [1978] considered a hormonal regulation because of the interdependence of adenylcyclase and cyclic AMP. Mees [1984] recently took up this theory again. Furthermore, Pike and Bosher [1980] identified furosemide as a potent inhibitor of the carboanhydrase in the stria vascularis. Other authors also discussed the potential importance of this enzyme for the ion transport in the stria vascularis [Erulkar and Maren, 1961; Watanabe and Ogawa, 1984]. The prostaglandins have also recently been held responsible for the edema formation in the stria vascularis after loop diuretic administration. Matthias [1984] documented the fulminant increase of the tissue prostaglandin concentration in the guinea pig's cochlea within a few minutes after furosemide administration.

The majority of the loop diuretic research on the stria vascularis was based on the hypothesis that the mechanism of effect of loop diuretics was the same for the inner ear as for the kidney. Since Burg and Green [1973], we know that the loop diuretics mainly cause diuresis by inhibition of the active chloride resorption in the ascending loop of Henle. We measured these chloride concentrations in the cochlear guinea pig endolymph after doses of EA which elicit the typical decline of the DC potential and strial edema (60 mg/kg body weight). However, these doses had no influence on the chloride concentration of 119 mmol. Therefore, the strial effect of EA cannot be related directly to its specific renal effect.

When considering Hapke's [1980] nomenclature of side effects by loop diuretics, the 'chloride experiment' must lead to the reevaluation of the term ototoxicity. Hapke proposed that a special organ toxicity of the loop diuretics could only be considered a specific effect when the same renal mechanism was present. Since the chloride concentration in the inner ear remained unchanged after EA application, an unspecific effect should be assumed here in any case.

Further indications of different modes of action in the kidney and inner ear were provided by the application of *l*-ozolinon. While changing the renal potassium concentration in the same way as EA, *l*-ozolinon did not change the endolymph potassium concentration in the inner ear of the guinea pig. However, the endolymphatic potential decreased at the same rapid rate as with EA. The obvious conclusion here is that the high endolymphatic potential in the mammalian cochlea is not directly connected with potassium activity.

The combination of *d*-ozolinon and EA also indicated a different mode of action of loop diuretics in the kidney and the inner ear. We have already stated that the nondiuretic ozolinon isomere antagonized the diuresis of furosemide and EA in the renal tubules [Greven and Heidenreich, 1980]. Our tests indicate that this renal competitive inhibition did not exist in the inner ear. The administration of *d*-ozolinon alone caused no decrease of the endolymphatic potential in the guinea pig cochlea, thus corresponding to the absence of renal diuresis. On the other hand, there was a rapid decline of the DC potential with the subsequent administration of 60 mg/kg body weight EA.

The lack of effect on the chloride transport and our results with the ozolinon isomere in the inner ear ruled out the term *specific* ototoxicity of loop diuretics in this instance too. Since the modes of action in the inner ear differ from the specific renal effects of these substances, we emphasize again that the unique sensitivity of the stria vascularis to loop diuretics is the product of the unspecific effects of these drugs.

Such unspecific effects following use of loop diuretics were also described for other organs with secretory epithelia. Knauf and Sachs [1980] observed similar effects in the salivary gland ducts of rats with different loop diuretics. These authors also found different modes of action here. Neither EA nor furosemide had an influence on the electrolyte transport and the electrical potential difference of these glandular epithelia. Using ozolinon, however, the sodium resorption and the potassium secretion were reduced. The potential difference remained unaffected. From this experiment it was concluded that there is no chloride and/or anion-dependent transport process at the ductal cell membrane of the salivary gland epithelia. The results of our chloride experiment in the inner ear led us to rule out a chloride-dependent transport mechanism as Knauf and Sachs [1980] has postulated for the rat's salivary glands.

The different modes of action of the loop diuretics in the kidney and the inner ear and the different effects in the cochlear and vestibular part of the guinea pig labyrinth and the whole inner ear of the pigeon demonstrate the uniqueness of the stria vascularis in the mammalian inner ear.

The uniqueness of the stria seems to be important for the regulation of the labyrinthine endolymph. We found that after EA application the characteristically rapid and fulminant functional changes of the mammalian cochlea occurred neither in the vestibular portion of the mammalian labyrinth nor in the whole pigeon labyrinth. This is in compliance with the fact that this unusually high potential of $+80$ mV for the whole organism was found only in the mammalian cochlear endolymph. All other labyrinthine portions investigated (vestibular in the guinea pig, cochlear and vestibular in the pigeon) had significantly lower potentials within the same narrow range. This is also true of potentials in labyrinths of other lower animal species, e.g. fish and reptiles [Schmidt, 1963; Enger, 1964; Rauch and Rauch, 1974].

Investigations into the postnatal morphological development of the stria vascularis are of particular interest with respect to the genesis of this uniquely high endolymphatic potential in the mammalian cochlea. It has been shown under the electron microscope that the stria vascularis is fully developed by the time the potential reaches $+20$ to $+80$ mV (between the 12th and 16th day) [Kikushi and Hilding, 1966; Bosher and Warren, 1971; Bosher, 1972]. The special structure of the stria vascularis seems to be the prerequisite for the development of high DC potential.

With the background of the different reactions of the stria vascularis and the tegmentum vasculosum in the pigeon to EA, the morphological details of the stria vascularis gain particular importance. With the scanning electron microscope examinations of the tegmentum vasculosum in the pigeon, we could demonstrate that the dark cells carry dense bushes of large microvilli. The light cells, however, are only sparsely covered by microvilli and, in addition, possess a centrally located kinocilium. The surface of the stria vascularis, however, is more similar to the light cells with their sparse covering of microvilli [Lim, 1969; Anniko, 1976; Horn et al., 1977; Cotanche and Salik, 1982]. Rauch and Reale [1964] found that the marginal cells lose their somewhat rudimentary kinocilia approximately on the 10th day postnatum. The tegmentum vasculosum in the pigeon appeared to be bordered by a basal membrane. Kikushi and Hilding [1966] could prove for the stria that the initially present basal membrane had involuted.

In summary, on comparing the species, one observes the following morphological picture of the different secretory labyrinth epithelia: the vestibular is the oldest portion of the labyrinth phylogenetically and does not change significantly as to its macroscopic and microscopic architecture through the ascending evolutional sequence to the mammalian [Werner,

1960; Baird, 1974; Fleischer, 1984]. From the lower vertebrates to the birds, the secretory epithelia in the cochlear portion of the labyrinth differ only slightly with a homogenous arrangement of light and dark cells [Kimura, 1931; Freye, 1952; Jahnke et al., 1969; Ishiyama et al., 1970]. The higher demands placed on the hearing apparatus of mammals are apparently fulfilled by a qualitative morphological change which is combined with improved functional features. The known morphological details of the stria vascularis develop further and the DC potential increases to $+80$ mV. The unique morphological structure of the stria vascularis, as compared with the vestibular apparatus of the labyrinth and the complete labyrinth of lower species, is not yet completely known. Engström et al. [1955] had noticed that the stria vascularis had a unique structure with seemingly 'intraepithelial' blood vessels. It was concluded that the intermediary cells must be mesenchymal elements and, therefore, only the marginal cells could be of epithelia origin. It has been proven since then, that the marginal cells are derived from the otocyst and that the intermediary cells are derived from the neural crest [Hilding and Ginsberg, 1977]. Because of the prominently large and dark pigment content of the intermediary cells, which is similar in appearance to that of the pigment in the vestibular part of the mammal labyrinth, one could discuss the possibility that the intermediary cells are actually a particular form of melanocyte [Kikushi and Hilding, 1966; Hilding and Ginsberg, 1977].

The ample supply of blood capillaries within the stria vascularis is the morphological prerequisite for the extremely high oxygen consumption which this epithel group needs in order to function. The oxygen consumption of the stria is even higher than that of the well perfused kidney [Chou, 1976]. Within the mammalian labyrinth, Chou and Rodgers [1979] found very different respiratory rates. The oxygen consumption was highest in the stria, with a value of 10.1 ml $O_2/100$ mg wet tissue/min (utricle wall 2.4, organ of Corti 0.9). A comparison of these values with those of other organs shows again the unique status of the stria vascularis. The respiratory rate in the liver is only 0.7, in the kidney in the proximal and distal tubules 3.6, in the collecting ducts only 0.8 and in the plexus chorioideus 5.6.

The high metabolic activity of the stria vascularis, coinciding with an ample blood supply, in contrast to the epithelia of the vestibular labyrinth, may be an essential cause of the different sensitivity of the two organ portions to loop diuretics. Bosher [1980] examined the EA effect in short intervals after administration of the drug. Initially after EA administration (3–5 min), there was shrinkage of the intermediary cells, first occurring immediately adjacent to the vessels. The swelling of the marginal cells could only be observed later. Other investigations also demonstrate to a primary obstruction of the strial blood capillaries 3 min after EA administration

[Akioyshi, 1981]. Orsulakova et al. [1981] also showed that the stria vascularis is particularly sensitive to anoxia. After an anoxia of 3 min duration, the ratio of sodium and potassium concentration was measured in the individual stria portions. In particular, in the area of the intermediary cells, the ratio of potassium to sodium had changed rapidly.

The good oxygen supply of the stria vascularis, however, cannot explain the different results in the cochlear and vestibular portion of the labyrinth, as the endolymphatic potential collapsed after administration of loop diuretics. From the classic experiment of Dohlmann and Radomski [1968], we know that even the relatively inconspicuous one-layered semi-circular canal epithelium is capable of a selective ion transport. This epithelium was capable of regaining the original potassium concentration in the endolymph after sodium chloride had been put into the semicircular canal. An assisting function of other epithelia could be excluded by bilateral clamping of the semicircular canal. In our experiments, neither morphological nor functional alterations occurred in the semicircular canal or in the ampulla after administration of EA. Similar results had been reported by Sellick and Johnstone [1974] with respect to the endolymphatic potential after intravenous administration of EA. In those experiments, EA was additionally applied locally to the endolymphatic space of the utricle. Although the ultricle potential could be suppressed to negative values, it did not decrease as rapidly and did not reach the same extreme negative values as in the cochlear endolymph, thus reflecting a different effect of EA on the stria.

The different reaction to EA of the different labyrinth portions leads to the assumption that, independent of the varying blood supply, there must be a special ion transport mechanism exclusively in the stria vascularis which is responsible for the high endolymphatic potential in this labyrinth portion.

In incomplete tests an effect similar to that seen by Sellick and Johnstone [1974] in the ampulla of the guinea pig occurred after local administration of EA in the pigeon. This local application caused a more significant decrease of the DC potential in the pigeon cochlea. This potential decreased even further when anoxic conditions were created by temporary nitrogen ventilation. These preliminary results contradict the above results for the mammalian cochlea [Vosteen, 1976]. The subsequent anoxia after EA in that study caused a re-increase of the endolymphatic potential.

If this potential decreasing effect of EA and anoxia appears in the mammalian vestibular organ and not, as shown by Vosteen [1976] in the cochlea, the final proof would be delivered for the hypothesis that there actually are different mechanisms of electrolyte transport in the different labyrinth portions.

In the future, loop diuretics will also be an indispensable component for investigations into the endolymph regulation, because they have proven to be of value for blocking the active ion transport systems. Basic research should be extended, with the next step being an analysis of the quantitative transfer of electrolytes through the membranes of the inner ear and measurement of intracellular ion concentrations.

5. Conclusions

Based on clinically observed hearing impairment and rare episodes of vertigo, both of which are well-known effects of glycoside administration, the loop diuretics have been classified as ototoxic.

In order to explore the specific mode of action of this drug category on the labyrinth, experiments were carried out on guinea pigs and pigeons. Light microscope, transmission and scanning electron microscope examinations served as morphologic criteria. The endolymphatic DC potential and the potassium, sodium and chloride concentrations in the endolymph were measured simultaneously as functional parameters. EA and the stereoisomeres of ozolinon were used as representative loop diuretics. The above experiments led to the following results:

(1) Unlike the damaging effects of aminoglycosides on the hair cells of the organ of Corti and the semicircular canal ampulla, the loop diuretics had a different site of attack in the inner ear. (a) Morphologically, subsequent to application of EA, an interstitial edema was observed between the intermediary cells of the stria vascularis and a hydrops of the marginal cells in the guinea pig. (b) Functionally, the edema correlated with a rapid decline of the endolymphatic potential from $+80$ mV to -40 mV with a simultaneous drop in the potassium and increase in the sodium concentrations in the endolymph. Both the morphological as well as the functional alterations were reversible.

(2) Under identical experimental conditions, the loop diuretics failed to create such an effect in the vestibular portion of the labyrinth in the guinea pigs and pigeons. There was no interstitial edema. The endolymphatic potential was affected very slowly and moderately. Therefore, the term 'ototoxicity' for loop diuretics must be restricted, since it is valid only with respect to the hearing portion and not with the vestibular apparatus of the inner ear.

(3) In pigeons, the secretory epithelia of the cochlea (tegmentum vasculosum) did not change following application of EA. There was neither interstitial edema nor functional alterations of the potential or electrolyte concentrations. Only sublethal drug doses led to substantial changes.

However, these are the results of a nonspecific overall toxic effect and do not represent a specific organ toxicity in the pigeon.

(4) Since the pigeon has no stria vascularis, and loop diuretics exclusively affect the stria vascularis of the mammalian cochlea, this drug group's effects should be called more precisely 'striatoxic', in contrast to the aminoglycosides which are 'ototoxic'.

(5) It was assumed for some time, that the loop diuretics affected the inner ear the same way as the kidney. The diuretic effect is mainly due to the inhibition of the active chloride absorption in the ascending loop of Henle. (a) In the guinea pig, the chloride concentration in the cochlear endolymph did not change following administration of EA. (b) *l*-Ozolinon led to a decrease of the potassium concentration in the kidney. The potassium concentration remained unchanged in the cochlear endolymph of the guinea pig after *l*-ozolinon. (c) The prior administration of the nondiuretic *d*-ozolinon leads to the competitive inhibition of the diuretic effect of the EA in the kidney. In contrast, in the guinea pig the effect of EA remained unchanged after injection of *d*-ozolinon.

(6) With respect to the mode of action of the loop diuretics on the stria vascularis, it may be concluded that this mechanism is a product of generalized effects, in other words effects that differ from the specific effect of these substances in the kidney.

(7) The unique reaction of the stria vascularis to the loop diuretics in comparison with other labyrinth areas seems to be of importance for the understanding of the endolymph production. In those parts of the labyrinth with a low endolymphatic potential (the complete pigeon labyrinth and the vestibular portion in the guinea pig), the loop diuretics did not cause functional alterations. Morphologically, there was no interstitial edema. This difference in behavior indicates that the stria vascularis alone possesses its own ion transport mechanism which can be blocked by the administration of loop diuretics. This particular function of the stria vascularis is probably responsible for the maintenance of the high DC potential of $+80 \, \mathrm{mV}$. This is unique in comparison with the far lower potential values in other portions of the endolymphatic space.

These results indicate that, in future times, the endolymph production for the different portions of the labyrinth (cochlea, ampulla, saccus endolymphaticus) must be examined more precisely. The postulate of different mechanisms for the endolymph production requires experimental verification.

Acknowledgements

The author expresses sincere gratitude to Prof. K.H. Vosteen (Director, ENT Department, University of Düsseldorf, FRG) for his generous support in all aspects of this study and for patient assistance. Special thanks are due to Prof. C. Morgenstern and Dr. O. Ninoyu who provided inestimably valuable advice in the electrophysiological experiments. Thanks also go to Mrs. R. Schwarzer (ENT Department) and Mrs. B. Jansen (Institute of Anatomy, University of Düsseldorf, Director: Prof. Rosenbauer) for the highly skilled production of the transmission and scanning electron micrographs.

Finally, the close collaboration of Mrs. O. Bull, Mrs. M. Janssen-Eiker and Mrs. M. Ahlrichs-Geising, who were responsible for the technical help, is appreciated.

References

Ahlström, P.; Thalmann, R.: Cyclic AMP and adenylcyclase in the inner ear. Laryngoscope 85: 1241 (1975).

Akiyoshi, M.: Effect of loop-diuretics on hair cells of the cochlea in guinea pigs. Histological and histochemical study. Scand. Audiol., suppl. 14, pp. 185–199 (1981).

Anniko, M.: Surface structure of stria vascularis in the guinea pig cochlea. Acta oto-lar. 82: 343–353 (1976).

Anniko, M.: Functional and morphological pathology of vestibular end organs. Revue de Laryngologie. 105: 205–216 (1984).

Anniko, M.; Bagger-Sjöbäck, D.: Early post mortem change of crista ampullaris. Virchows Arch. Abt. B Zellpath. 25: 137–149 (1977).

Anniko, M.; Sarkady, L.: The effects of mercurial poisoning on the vestibular system. Acta oto-lar. 85: 96–104 (1978).

Anniko, M.; Spångberg, M.-L.; Schacht, J.: Adenylate cyclase activity in the fetal and early postnatal inner ear of the mouse. Hear. Res. 4: 11–22 (1981).

Aran, J.-M.; Sauvage, C. de: Evolution of CM, SP, AP during ethacrynic acid intoxication in the guinea pig. Acta oto-lar. 83: 153–159 (1977).

Arnold, W.; Morgenstern, C.; Thorn, L.; Schinko, I.: Morphologische und funktionelle Veränderungen am Innenohr nach Vergiftung mit Etacrynsäure und Atoxyl. Archs Oto-Rhino-Lar. 218: 179–190 (1978).

Arnold, W.; Nadol, J.B.; Weidauer, H.: Temporal bone histopathology in human ototoxicity due to loop diuretics. Scand. Audiol., suppl. 14, pp. 201–213 (1981).

Bagger-Sjöback, D.; Filipek, C.S.; Schacht, J.: Characteristics and drug responses of cochlear and vestibular adenylate cyclase. Archs Oto-Rhino-Lar. 228: 217–222 (1980).

Baird, I.L.: Anatomical features of the inner ear in submammalian vertebrates. Handbook of sensory physiology, sect. V/1, pp. 179–212 (Springer, Berlin 1974).

Békésy, G. von: DC resting potentials inside the cochlear partition. J. acoust. Soc. Am. 24: 72–76 (1952).

Bosher, S.K.: Neonatal changes in the endolymph and their possible relationship to the peri-natal deafness. Acta oto-lar. 73: 203–211 (1972).

Bosher, S.K.: The nature of the negative endocochlear potentials produced by anoxia and ethacrynic acid in the rat and guinea pig. J. Physiol. 293: 329–345 (1979).

Bosher, S.K.: The nature of the ototoxic actions of ethacrynic acid upon the mammalian endolymph system. II. Structural-functional correlates in the stria vascularis. Acta oto-lar. 90: 40–54 (1980).

Bosher, S.K.; Smith, C.; Warren, R.L.: The effects of ethacrynic acid upon the cochlear endolymph and stria vascularis. A preliminary report. Acta oto-lar. *75:* 184–191 (1973).

Bosher, S.K.: Warren, R.L.: A study of the electrochemistry and osmotic relationships of the cochlear fluids in the neonatal rat at the time of the development of the endocochlear potential. J. Physiol. *212:* 739–761 (1971).

Breschet, G.: Recherches anatomiques et physiologiques sur l'organe de l'ouie dans les oiseaux; in Ann. des Sciences Naturelles, partie zoologique, sec. série, vol. 5, Paris (1836).

Brown, H.; Hinshu, H.: Toxic reaction of streptomycin on the eight nerve apparatus. Proc. Mayo Clin. *21:* 347 (1946).

Brown, R.D.: Comparison of the cochlear toxicity of sodium ethacrynate, furosemide and cysteine adduction of sodium ethacrynate in cats. Toxicol. appl. Pharmacol. *31:* 270–282 (1975).

Brown, R.D.; McElwee, J.R.: Effects of intra-arterially and intra-venously administered ethacrynic acid and furosemide on cochlear N_1 in cats. Toxicol. appl. Pharmacol. *22:* 589–594 (1972).

Brummet, R.; Smith, C.A.; Veno, Y.; Cameron, S.; Richter, R.: The delayed effects of ethacrynic acid on the stria vascularis of guinea pig. Acta oto-lar. *83:* 98–112 (1977).

Brummet, R.; Traynor, J.; Brown, R.; Himes, D.: Cochlear damage resulting from kanamycin and furosemide. Acta oto-lar. *80:* 86 (1975).

Burg, M.; Green, N.: Effect of ethacrynic acid on the thick ascend limb of Henle's loop. Kidney int. *4:* 301–308 (1973).

Case, D.B.; Gunther, S.J.; Cannon, P.J.: Ethacrynate-induced depression of respiration in transport systems and kidney mitochrondria. Am. J. Physiol. *224:* 769 (1973).

Causse, R.: Action toxique vestibulaire et cochléaire de la streptomycine au point de vue expérimental. Annls Oto-lar. *66:* 518 (1949).

Causse, R.; Gondet, I.; Vallancien, B.: Action de la streptomycine sur les cellules ciliées des organes vestibulaires de la souris. C.r. Séanc. Soc. Biol. *143:* 619–620 (1949).

Chou, J.T.Y.: Respiration of tissues lining the mammalian membranous labyrinth. J. Laryngol. *76:* 341 (1976).

Chou, J.T.Y.; Rodgers, K.: Respirationsraten der Wandstrukturen des membranösen Labyrinths beim Meerschweinchen im Vergleich mit anderen Körpergeweben; cited by Arnold, W.; Vosteen, K.H.: Physiologie von Perilymphe und Endolymphe, Hals-, Nasen-, Obrenheilkunde in Praxis und Klinik, Bd 5 (Thieme, Stuttgart 1979).

Citron, L.; Exley, D.: Recent work on the biochemistry of the labyrinthine fluids. Proc. R. Soc. Med. *50:* 697–701 (1957).

Civan, M.M.: Intracellular activities of sodium and potassium. Am. J. Physiol. *234:* 261–269 (1978).

Cotanche, D.A.; Sulik, K.K.: Scanning electron microscopy of the developing chick tegmentum vasculosum. Scann. Electron Microsc. *III:* 1283–1294 (1982).

Dohlman, G.F.: Secretion and absorption of endolymph. Annls Oto-lar. *73:* 708–723 (1964).

Dohlman, G.F.: Investigations on the presence of acid Mucopolysaccharides in the endolymph of pigeons. Proc. Barany Soc. (1970).

Dohlman, G.F.: Critical review of the concept of cupula function. Acta oto-lar., suppl. 376 (1980).

Dohlman, G.F.; Boord, R.: The effects of cupular removal on the activity of ampullary structures in the pigeon. Acta oto-lar. *57:* 507–516 (1965).

Dohlman, G.F.; Radomski, M.W.: The ion selective function of the epithelium of the membraneous canal walls. Acta oto-lar. *66:* 409–416 (1968).

Duvall, A.J.; Quick, C.A.: Tracers and endogenous debris in delineating cochlear barriers and pathways. Annls Oto-lar. *78:* 1041–1057 (1969).

Duvall, A.J.; Santi, P.A.; Hukee, M.J.: Cochlear fluid balance – a clinical research overview. Ann. Otol. Rhinol. Lar. *89:* 335–341 (1980).

Duvall, A.J.; Wersall, J.: Site of action of streptomycin upon inner ear sensory cells. Acta oto-lar. *57:* 581–598 (1964).

Enger, P.S.: Ionic composition of the cranial and labyrinthine fluids and sacculor DC potentials in fish. Compar. Biochem. Physiol. *11:* 131–137 (1964).

Engström, H. Sjöstrand, F.S.; Spöndlin, H.: Feinstruktur der Stria vascularis beim Meerschweinchen. Pract. Oto. Rhino. Laryng. *17:* 69–79 (1955).

Ernstson, S.: Ethacrynic acid-induced hearing loss in guinea pigs. Acta oto-lar. *73:* 476 (1972).

Erulkar, S.D.; Maren, T.H.: Carbonic anhydrase and the inner ear. Nature *189:* 459–460 (1961).

Falk, S.A.: Combined effects of noise and ototoxic drugs. Environ. Health Perspect. *2:* 5 (1972).

Farrington, R.; Hull-Smith, H., Bunn, P.; McDermott, W.: Streptomycin toxicity. Reactions to highly purified drug on long-continued administration to human subjects. J. Am. med. Ass. *34:* 679 (1947).

Fleischer, G.: Geschichte des Ohres – Geschichte der Erde. HNO *2:* 7–23 (1984).

Forge, A.: Observations on the stria vascularis of the guinea pig cochlea and the changes resulting from the administration of the diuretic furosemide. Clin. Otolaryngol. *1:* 211 (1976).

Freye, H.-A.: Das Gehörorgan der Vögel. Wiss. Z. Martin-Luther-Univers. Halle-Wittenberg *5:* Jahrgang II (1952/53).

Gomolin, I.H.; Garshik, E.: Ethacryn acid induced deafness accompanied by nystagmus. New Engl. J. Med. *Sept.:* 80 (1980).

Greven, J.; Beckers, M.; Defrain, W.; Meywald, K.; Heidenreich, O.: Studies with the optically active isomers of the new diuretic drug ozolinone. II. Inhibition by *d*-ozolinone of furosemide-induced diuresis. Pflügers Arch. *384:* 61–64 (1980a).

Greven, J.; Defrain, W.; Glaser, K.; Meywald, K.; Heidenreich, O.: Studies with the optically active isomers of the new diuretic drug ozolinone. I. Differences in stereoselectivity of the renal target structures of ozolinone. Pflügers Arch. *384:* 57–60 (1980b).

Greven, J.; Heidenreich, O.: Effects of ozolinone, a diuretic active metabolite of etozolinone, on renal function. I. Clearance studies in dogs. Archs Pharmacol. *304:* 283–287 (1978).

Greven, J.; Heidenreich, O.: Zur Frage der Stereospezifität von Diuretikawirkungen anhand des Beispiels von Ozolinon; in Diuretika, edition Medizin (Weinheim, Deerfield Beach 1980).

Greven, J.; Klein, H.; Heidenreich, O.: Effects of ozolinone, a diuretic active metabolite of etozolinone, on renal function. II. Localisation of tubular site of diuretic action by micropuncture in the rat. Archs Pharmacol. *304:* 289–296 (1978).

Guild, St.R.: Circulation of the endolymph. Am. J. Anat. *39:* 57–68 (1927).

Hallpike, C.S.; Cairns, H.: Observations on the pathology of Ménière's syndrome. J. Lar. Otol. *53:* 625–655 (1938).

Hapke, H.-J.: Vergleichende Toxikologie der Diuretika; in Rosenthal, Knauf, Diuretika. Workshop, Lissabon 1979, edition Medizin (Weinheim, Deerfield Beach 1980).

Haubrich, J.; Schätzle, W.: Zur Frage histochemischer Veränderungen der Meerschweinchenschnecke unter dem Einfluss von Diuretika. Arch. klin. exp. Ohr.-Nas.-KehlkHeilk. *196:* 319 (1970).

Haubrich, J.; Schätzle, W.: Histochemische Veränderungen der Meerschweinchenschnecke unter dem experimentellen Einfluss des Diuretikums Hydromedin. Arch. klin. exp. Ohr.-Nas.-KehlkHeilk. *199:* 595 (1971).

Helmchen, U.; Fischbach, H.; Schmidt, U.: Akute Schäden des proximalen Tubulusepithels der Rattenniere nach einer einmaligen hochdosierten Furosemidgabe. Klin. Wschr. *49:* 1298 (1971).

Hilding, D.A.: Cochlear chromaffin cells. Laryngoscope *75:* 1–15 (1965).

Hilding, D.A.; Ginsberg, R.D.: Pigmentation of the stria vascularis. Acta oto-lar. *84:* 24–37 (1977).

Hiraide, F.: The histochemistry of dark cells in the vestibular labyrinth. Acta oto-lar *71:* 40–48 (1971).

Hommerich, C.P.: Morphologische Befunde am sekretorischen Epithel der Ampulle nach Etacrynsäure. Laryngol. Rhinol. Otol. *64:* 209–213 (1985).

Horn, K.L.; Ende, M.J.; Langley, L.R.; Gates, G.A.: Scanning ultrastructure of the stria vascularis. Archs Oto-Rhino-Lar. *215:* 35–43 (1977).

Igarashi, M.; Yoshinobu, T.: Comparative observations of the eminentia cruciata in birds and mammals. Anat. Rec. *155:* 269–277 (1966).

Ishiyama, E.; Cutt, R.A.; Keels, E.W.: Ultrastructure of the tegmentum vasculosum and transitional zone. Ann. Otol. *79:* 998–1009 (1970).

Ishiyama, E.; Keels, E.W.: New morphological aspects of the horizontal crista in pigeon. Acta anat. *79:* 1–14 (1971).

Jahnke, V.; Lundquist, P.-G.; Wersäll, J.: Some morphological aspects of sound perception in birds. Acta oto-lar. *67:* 583–601 (1969).

Johnstone, C.G.; Schmidt, R.S.; Johnstone, B.M.: Sodium and potassium in vertebrate cochlear endolymph as determined by flame microspectrometry. Compar. Biochem. Physiol. *9:* 335–341 (1963).

Jörgensen, F.O.: Cochlear potentials of the pigeon inner ear recorded with microelectrodes. Acta physiol. scand. *100:* 393–403 (1977).

Jung, W.; Rosskopf, K.: Evoked Response Audiometry (ERA) am Meerschweinchen vor und nach Lasix-induziertem Hörverlust. Lar. Rhinol. Otol. *54:* 411 (1975).

Kerr, T.P.; Ross, M.D.; Ernst, S.A.: Cellular localisation of Na^+, K^+-ATP-ase in the mammalian cochlear duct: significance for cochlear fluid balance. Am. J. Otolaryngol. *3:* 332–338 (1982).

Kikushi, K.; Hilding, D.A.: The development of the stria vascularis in the mouse. Acta oto-lar. *62:* 277–291 (1966).

Kimura, R.S.: Distribution, structure and function of dark cells in the vestibular labyrinth. Annls Oto-lar. *78:* 542–560 (1969).

Kimura, R.S.; Lundquist, P.-G.; Wersäll, J.: Secretory epithelial linings in the ampullae of the guinea pig labyrinth. Acta oto-lar. *57:* 517–530 (1964).

Kimura, R.S.; Schuknecht, H.F.: The ultrastructure of the human stria vascularis. I. Acta oto-lar. *69:* 415–427 (1970).

Kimura, T.: Morphologische Untersuchungen über das membranöse Gehörorgan der Vögel. Folia anat. jap. *9:* 91–142 (1931).

Knauf, H.; Sachs, G.: Modelluntersuchungen zum Wirkungsmechanismus von Diuretika; in Diuretika, edition Medizin (Weinheim, Deerfield Beach 1980).

Kohonen, A.; Janhidinen, T.; Tarkkanen, J.: Experimental deafness caused by ethacrynic acid. Acta oto-lar. *70:* 187–189 (1970).

Komnick, H.; Komnick, U.: Elektronenmikroskopische Untersuchungen zur funktionellen Morphologie des Ionentransportes in der Salzdrüse von *Larus argentatus.* Z. Zellforsch. *60:* 163–203 (1963).

Konishi, T.; Mendelssohn, M.: Effect of ouabain on cochlear potentials and endolymph composition in guinea pigs. Acta oto-lar. *69:* 192 (1970).

Kregenow, F.M.: Cell volume control in water relations in membrane transport in plants and animals; in Jungreis et al. Current topics in membranes and transport, vol. 9, p. 291 (Academic Press, New York 1977).

Kockenthal, W.; Matthes, E.; Renner, M.: Leitfaden für das zoologische Praktikum (Fischer, Stuttgart 1971).

Kuijpers, W.: Cation transport and cochlear function. Acta oto-lar. *67:* 200–205 (1969).

Kuijpers, W.; Bonting, S.L.: The nature of the cochlear endolymphatic resting potential. Pflügers Arch. *320:* 359–372 (1970).

Kuijpers, W.; Vleuten, A.C. van der; Bonting, S.L.: Cochlear function and sodium and potassium activated adenosine triphosphate. Science *157:* 949–950 (1967).

Kuijpers, W.; Wilberts, D.P.C.: The effect of ouabain and ethacrynic acid on ATP-ase activities in the inner ear of the rat and guinea pig. ORL *38:* 321–327 (1976).

Kurz, H.; Neumann, H.-G.: Wirkungen von Pharmaka auf den Organismus; in Forth, Henschler, Rummel, Allgemeine und spezielle Pharmakologie und Toxikologie (Wissenschaftsverlag, Bibliographisches Institut, Mannheim 1977).

Kusakari, J.; Ise, I.; Comegys, J.H.; Thalmann, I.; Thalmann, R.: Effect of ethacrynic acid, furosemide and oubain upon the endolymphatic potential and upon high energy phosphates of stria vascularis. Laryngoscope *88:* 12–37 (1978).

Kusakari, J.; Sato, Y.; Kobayashi, T.; Saijo, S.; Kawamoto, K.: Effect of ethacrynic acid upon the peripheral vestibular nystagmus. Adv. Oto-Rhino-Laryng., vol. 25, pp. 1178–183 (Karger, Basel 1979).

Kusakari, J.; Thalmann, R.: Effects of anoxia and ethacrynic acid upon ampullar potential and upon high energy phosphates in ampullar wall. Laryngoscope *86:* 132–147 (1976).

Lagarriga, J.; Buenrrostro, C.; Rodriguez, P.; Castaneda, J.: Hepatonecrosis caused by furosemide. Special lesions of various species? Rev. Gastroenterol. Mex. *42:* 117 (1977).

Lehnhardt, E.: Klinik der Innenohrschwerhörigkeiten. Archs Oto-Rhino-Lar., suppl., 58–218 (1984).

Levinson, R.M.; Capps, M.J.; Mathog, R.H.: Ethacrynic acid, furosemide and vestibular caloric responses. Annls Oto-lar. *83:* 223–229 (1974).

Lim, D.J.: Three-dimensional observation of the inner ear with the scanning electron microscope. Acta oto-lar., suppl. 255 (1969).

Lim, D.J.: Vestibular sensory organs. A scanning electron microscopic investigation. Archs Oto-lar. *94:* 69–76 (1971).

Lim, D.J.; Freilich, I.W.: Ultrastructure of the stria vascularis, vestibular dark cells and endolymphatic sac following acute diuretic ototoxicity. Scand. Audiol. *14:* suppl. pp. 139–155 (1981).

Maher, J.F.; Schreiner, G.E.: Studies on ethacrynic acid on patients with refractory edema. Ann. intern. Med. *62:* 15 (1965).

Marumo, F.; Mishinat, I.: Effects of ethacrynic acid and furosemide on the hormon-mediated adenylate-cyclase activation of the hamster kidney. Endocr. jap. *25:* 423–430 (1978).

Mathog, R.H.: Vestibulototoxicity of ethacrynic acid. Laryngoscope *87:* 1791–1808 (1977).

Mathog, R.H.; Capps, M.J.: Ototoxic interactions of ethacrynic acid and streptomycin. Annls Oto-lar. *86:* 158–163 (1977).

Mathog, R.H.; Thomas, W.H.; Hudson, W.R.: Ototoxicity of new potent diuretic. Archs Oto-lar. *92:* 7 (1970).

Matschinsky, F.M.; Thalmann, R.: Energy metabolism of the cochlear duct; in Paparella, Biochemical mechanism in hearing and deafness, pp. 265–294 (Thomas Springfield 1970).

Matthias, R.: Einfluss der Prostaglandine auf die Diuretika-Ototoxizität. Arch. Ohr.-Nas.-KehlkHeilk., suppl., pp. 83–85 (1984).

Matz, G.J.: The ototoxic effects of ethacrynic acid in man and animals. Laryngoscope *86:* 1065–1086 (1976).

Matz, G.J.; Naunton, R.F.: Ototoxic drugs and poor renal function. J. Am. med. Ass. *206:* 2119 (1968).

McCurdy, J.A.; McCormick, J.G.: Ototoxicity of ethacrynic acid in the anuric guinea pig. Archs. Oto-lar. *100:* 143 (1974).

McNight, A.D.C.; Leaf, A.: Regulation of cellular volume. Physiol. Rev. *57:* 510 (1977).

Mees, K.: Ultrastructural localization of K^+-dependent, oubain sensitive NPP-ase (Na-K-ATP-ase) in the guinea pig inner ear. Acta oto-lar. *95:* 277 (1983).

Mees, K.: Die hormonelle Steuerung des Innenohres. Laryngol. Rhinol. Otol. *63:* 626–632 (1984).

Meyer zum Gottesberge-Orsulakova, A.: Pigment und Ionentransport im Vestibularorgan. Arch. Ohr.-nas.- KehlkHelik., suppl., pp. 75–76 (1984).

Meyer zum Gottesberge-Orsulakova, A.: Melanin in the inner ear: micromorphological and microanalytical investigation. Acta histochem. *102:* 222–272 (1986).

Molitor, H.; Graessle, O.E.; Kuna, S.; Mushett, C.W.; Silber, R.H.: Some toxicological and pharmacological properties of streptomycin. J. Pharmac. exp. Ther. *98:* 151–173 (1946).

Morgenstern, C.; Lessmann, F.J.; Amano, H.; Orsulakova, A.; Juhn, S.K.: Inner ear effects of a new loop diuretic (Ozolinon). Scand. Audiol., *14:* suppl., pp. 111–118 (1981).

Naftalin, L.; Harrison, M.S.: Circulation of labyrinthine fluids. J. Laryngol. *72:* 118–136 (1958).

Nakai, Y.: Electron microscopic study of the inner ear after ethacrynic acid intoxication. Practica oto-rhino-lar. *33:* 366–376 (1971).

Nakai, Y.; Hilding, D.A.: Electron microscopic studies of adenosine triphosphatase activity in the stria vascularis and spiral ligament. Acta oto lar. *62:* 411–428 (1966).

Nakai, Y.; Hilding, D.A.: Adenosine triphosphatase distribution in the organ of Corti. Acta oto-lar. *64:* 477–491 (1967).

Necker, R.: Zur Entstehung der Cochleapotentiale von Vögeln: Verhalten bei O_2-Mangel, Cyanidvergiftung und Unterkühlung sowie Beobachtungen über die räumliche Verteilung. Z. vergl. Physiol. *69:* 367–425 (1970).

Ninoyu, O.; Hommerich, C.P.; Morgenstern, C.: Zur Ototoxizität von Schleifendiuretika. Archs. Oto-Rhino-Lar., suppl. 1985/2.

Novikoff, A.B.: Lysosomes in the physiology and pathology of cells: contributions of staining methods. Ciba Fdn Symp., pp. 36–77 (1963).

Orsulakova, A.; Kaufmann, R.; Morgenstern, C.; D'Haese, M.: Cation distribution of the cochlea wall (stria vascularis). Fresenius Z. Anal. Chem. *308:* 221–223 (1981).

Othani, J.; Ohtsuki, K.; Omata, T.; Ouchi, J.; Saito, T.: Potentiation and its mechanism of cochlear damage resulting from furosemide and aminoglycoside antibiotics. ORL *40:* 53 (1978).

Paloheimo, S.; Thalmann, R.: Influence of 'loop' diuretics upon Na^+/K^+-ATP-ase and adenylate cyclase of the stria vascularis. Archs Oto-Rhino-Lar. *217:* 347–359 (1977).

Pike, D.A.; Bosher, S.K.: The time course of strial changes produced by intravenous furosemide. Hear. Res. *3:* 79–89 (1980).

Post, R.L.; Merrit, C.R.; Kinsolving, C.R.: Membrane adenosine triphosphatase as a participant in the active transport of sodium and potassium in the human erythrocyte. J. biol. Chem. *235:* 1796–1802 (1960).

Prazma, J.; Browder, J.; Fischer, N.D.: Ethacrynic acid ototoxicity potentation by kanamycin. Ann. Otol. Rhinol. Lar. *83:* 11 (1974).

Prazma, J.; Thomas, W.G.; Fischer, N.O.; Preslar, M.J.: Ototoxicity of the ethacrynic acid. Archs Oto-lar. *95:* 448 (1972).

Quick, C.A.; Duvall, A.J.: Early changes in the cochlear duct from ethacrynic acid: an electronmicroscopic evaluation. Laryngoscope *80:* 945–965 (1970).

Rauch, S.; Rauch, I.: Physico-chemical properties of the inner ear especially ionic transport; in Keidel, Neff, Handbook of sensory, pp. 647–682 (Springer, Berlin 1974).

Richet, G.; Hagege, J.: Dark cells of the distal convoluted tubules and collectining ducts. II. Physiological significance. Fortschr. Zool. *23:* 299 (1975).

Ross, M.D.; Ernst, S.A.; Kerr, T.P.: Possible functional roles of Na$^+$, K$^+$-ATP-ase in the inner ear and their relevance to Ménière's disease. Am. J. Otolaryngol. *3:* 353–360 (1982).

Rüedi, C.; Furrer, W.; Lüthy, F.; Nager, G.; Tschirren, B.: Further observations concerning the toxic effects of streptomycin and quinine on the auditory organ of guinea pigs. Laryngoscope *62:* 333 (1952).

Satzinger, G.; Herrmann, M.; Vollmer, K.-O.; Merzweiler, A.; Gomahr, H.; Heidenreich, O.; Greven, J.: Etozolinon: a novel diuretic; in Cragoe, Diuretic agents, p. 155 Chemical Society, Washington 1978).

Schacht, J.: Adenylate cyclase and cochlear fluid balance. Am. J. Otolaryngol. *3:* 328–331 (1982).

Schermuly, L.; Göttl, K.H.; Klinke, R.: Little ototoxic effect of furosemide on the pigeon inner ear. Hear. Res. *10:* 279–282 (1983).

Schmidt, R.S.: Types of endolymphatic potentials. Compar. Biochem. Physiol. *10:* 83–88 (1963).

Schmidt, R.S.; Fernandez, J.: Labyrinthine DC potentials in representative vertebrates. J. cell. comp. Physiol. *59:* 311–322 (1962).

Schneider, W.J.; Becker, E.L.: Acute transient hearing loss after ethacrynic acid therapy. Archs intern. Med. *117:* 715–717 (1966).

Schwarz, F.D.; Pillay, V.K.G.; Kark, R.M.: Ethacrynic acid: its useful and untoward effects. Am. Heart J. *79:* 427–428 (1970).

Sellick, P.M.; Johnstone, B.M.: Differential effects of oubain and ethacrynic acid on the labyrinthine potentials. Pflügers Arch. *352:* 229 (1974).

Shambaugh, G.E.: Über die Herkunft der in den tieferen Schichten der Stria vascularis sich findenden Zellen. Z. Ohrenheilk. *53:* 312 (1907).

Shambaugh, G., Jr.; Derlacki, E.; Harrison, W.; House, H.; House, W.; Hildyard, V.; Schuknecht, H.; Shea, J.: Dihydrostreptomycin deafness. J. Am. med. Ass. *170:* 1657 (1959).

Silverstein, H.; Begin, R.: Ethacrynic acid – its reversible ototoxicity. Laryngoscope *84:* 976 (1974).

Skou, J.C.: Enzymatic basis for active transport of Na$^+$ and K$^+$ across cell membrane. Physiol. Rev. *45:* 596–617 (1965).

Smith, C.A.: Structure of the stria vascularis and the spiral prominence. Annls Oto-lar. *66:* 521–536 (1957).

Smith, C.A.; Lowry, O.H.; Wu, M.L.: The electrolytes of the labyrinthine fluids. Laryngoscope *66:* 141–153 (1954).

Spöndlin, H.: Zur Ototoxizität des Streptomycins. Practica oto-rhino-lar. *28:* 305–322 (1966).

Syka, J.; Melichar, I.: Comparison of the effects of furosemide and ethacrynic acid upon the cochlear function in the guinea pig. Scand. Audiol., suppl. 14, pp. 63–69 (1981).

Tasaki, I.; Davis, H.; Eldredge, D.H.: Exploration of cochlear potentials in guinea pig with a micro-electrode. J. acoust. Soc. Am. *26:* 765–773 (1954)

Vargish, T.; Benjamin, R.; Shenkman, L.: Deafness from furosemide. Ann. intern. Med. *73:* 761 (1970).

Vosteen, K.H.: Neue Aspekte zur Biologie und Pathologie des Innenohres. Arch. Ohr.-Nas.-KehlkHelik. *178:* 1–104 (1961).

Vosteen, K.H.: Die Produktion von Endo- und Perilymphe und die Durchlässigkeit von Innenohrmembranen. Archs Oto-Rhino-Lar. *212:* 211–221 (1976).

Watanabe, K.; Ogawa, A.: Carbonic anhydrase activity in stria vascularis and dark cells in vestibular labyrinth. Ann. Otol. Rhinol. Lar. *93:* 262–266 (1984).

Werner, C.F.: Das Gehörorgan der Wirbeltiere und des Menschen. Beispiel für eine vergleichende Morphologie der Lagebeziehungen (Thieme, Leipzig 1960).

Wersäll, J.: Studies on the structure and innervation of the sensory epithelium of the ampulla in the guinea pig. Acta oto-lar., suppl. 126 (1956).

Wersäll, J.; Björkroth, B.; Flock, Å.; Lundquist, P.-G.: Experiments on ototoxic effects of antibiotics. Fortschr. Hals- Nas.-Ohrenheilk., vol. 20, pp. 14–41 (Karger, Basel 1973).

West, B.A.; Brummet, R.E.; Himes, D.L.: Interaction of kanamycin and ethacrynic acid. Severe cochlear damage in guinea pigs. Archs Oto-lar. *98:* 32 (1973).

Wit, H.P.; Bleeker, J.D.: The effect of ototoxic agents and anoxia upon the second-evoked vestibular whole nerve action potential. 19th Workshop on Inner Ear Biology, Mainz 1982.

Wolff, D.: Melanin in the inner ear. Archs Oto-lar. *14:* 195–211 (1931).

Christian Peter Hommerich, MD, ENT-Clinic, University of Düsseldorf,
D-4000 Düsseldorf (FRG)

Subject Index